D1234867

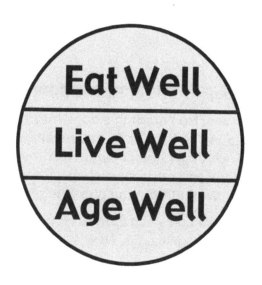

Eat Well
Live Well
Age Well

Patricia Greenberg

Published by The Fitness Gourmet
Los Angeles, CA, New York, NY

Printed in the United States of America

Design by BGFA

Library of Congress Cataloging-in-Publication Data
Greenberg, Patricia
Eat Well, Live Well, Age Well

ISBN-13: 978-0578602721
ISBN-10: 0578602725

Acknowledgements

Writing this book was, to date, my most challenging project. It took 18 years of intense research, following the lives of everyone around me, witnessing astonishing changes in the world, studying science and history, reading about the latest developments in nutrition and fitness related to aging, and dealing with the ups and downs of my own life as it continues to unfold. I spent countless hours agonizing over what to say and how to say it, knowing at some point I had to organize the information and put it to paper.

The big questions that needed answers were always circling back to the meaning of life, how eating well and living well help us age well, and how profound it is that some people die young and others seem to live well beyond their life expectancy. Well, that is life, there are no guarantees, no single path, and no one gets out alive. What I have learned and what I am so happy to share, is that you have the power to control your own happiness and quality of life for the rest of your days. I want to thank all those who have helped me bring this book to fruition and make living and aging worthwhile.

I want to start out by giving thanks to my husband, Aaron Grunfeld, whom I love very much for giving me the freedom and support necessary to embark on this incredible journey. I look forward to many more years of healthy aging together! To my daughter, Gabriella Grunfeld, who makes me laugh and smile everyday with her youthful optimism and inexhaustible curiosity for learning in everything she does. To my cousin, Livia Salamon, who spent countless hours with me sharing her musings about aging and her invaluable feedback on each chapter as it unfolded, thank you for listening.

To my writing partner, Denise Hidalgo, who won't take anywhere near the credit she deserves. She made this book happen, taking my scrappy notes and rambling emails and forming them into a cohesive and intelligent manuscript. I would not have been able to do this without her! To BGFA, for the design and layout of the book, making it more beautiful that I could have imagined possible. To Cheri Lasher for her brilliant artistic eye designing the cover, her talent never ceases to amaze me.

Lastly and most importantly to my four fabulous siblings, Elizabeth Greenberg, Bert Green, Steve Greenberg, and Janice Horowitz. We have been through all of life's triumphs and tribulations together, both happy and sad, and will continue to stay together as a unified force forever.

Introduction

Eat Well, Live Well, Age Well. I wrote this book for myself as much as for you, the reader. Even though our personal experiences may be very different, I really believe we are all in this together. A community of people well into adulthood who want to pursue wellness and happiness for the rest of our lives. I am 58 now and have been working on this project since I turned 40. At that time I saw so many people my age who were terrified to be moving out of their thirties, and yet I felt so young and vibrant. I got married at 37, my career was going strong, and at 40 I had a beautiful new daughter. I was running long distance road races on a regular basis, writing books and speaking all over the country on eating well and living well. And yet more and more I was hearing, you need to slow down, it's not appropriate for a woman over 40 to be running around in spandex pants, why do you run, you're almost 50, don't your knees hurt? You get the picture.

It was even worse when these remarks came from family and friends, because I came to my successes later in life than most, and they were not accustomed to seeing me at my peak physically, mentally and emotionally. While my siblings were slender and athletic, I was a chubby child and teen, and one of the high school nicknames I had to endure was "Fatty Patty." Thirty years later, I finally found my stride and yet I was still being knocked down, or at least that's how it felt. In reality, I think that like many of us, I had bought into the concept that we all slow down as we age, that we are not as agile, strong, emotionally sound, attractive, capable, etc., as when we were younger, and those expectations cause us to treat each other — and ourselves — as if those things were true, even if they are not.

"Act Your Age — there are no right or wrong things to do at any age!"

During my late 40s and into my mid-50s, I cut back to part-time work and stayed close to home to care for my family. With loved ones more than a decade older than I was, issues relating to healthy aging took a real priority for me, especially when I had to cope with a series of unexpected and painful losses within a short span of time. I saw many of my friends and family, both professionally and personally, making decisions based on what they thought they "should" be doing at their age: they stopped doing what they loved based on pre-conceived notions about what is age appropriate. Like many self-fulfilling prophecies, what we expect as we grow older, we can make come to pass — but the reverse is also true, so with a little effort and the idea that "age is nothing but a number," we can keep youthful health and glow long into our advanced years. *I almost named this book "Act your Age," because I wanted to address this idea — that there are no right or wrong things to do at any age!*

As the years went by, I started experiencing a number of rejections for work opportunities based on my age, sight unseen. I found that infuriating, and yet it seemed that there was nothing I could do about it. It finally hit me why so many people were lying about their age, knocking off up to 10 years of experience from their resumes. The concept of empowering people as we age didn't even exist 10 years ago, and 20 years ago people were forced to retire with no means of fighting back. The devastating emotions that my friends, family members, and colleagues were experiencing as they faced this kind of baseless age discrimination is what first sparked my interest and sent me on the journey of learning about how and why we age. This became my driving motivation in life, and in the creation of this book.

I spent a lot of time researching how age affects us, how people perceive each other (and themselves) as we age, how even our best friends and closest family members value and view older people, and what to do at different stages of our lives to ensure vibrant health. And yet, what I learned through my research and observation seemed incongruent with how I was actually living my own life. Everyone seemed then — and to a significant degree, now — to be terrified of getting old. As all of this was swirling around in my head, it never occurred to me that I was aging, too.

I would like people of all ages to understand and embrace how and why we age, providing strategies to help each of us live life to the fullest as we move on in years. One of the greatest accomplishments in life is to accept the things you cannot change — while still doing something about the things you can change, before it's too late. I want to convey from personal experience that there is no such thing as "anti-aging" — there are no miracle creams or cures to turn back time. Cosmetic procedures such as fillers, Botox and even cosmetic surgery may be an option to feel better about how you look, but nothing stops time from moving forward. Trust me, I have tried them all! Living well is the only way to survive and endure the aging process. Growing older is inevitable, but we can learn to embrace it, and make every day of our lives wonderful by developing lifestyle habits that work, and planning ahead helps us to feel more in control and reduce stress in regard to aging.

"Stay In Today"

I also found that whether you have a lot of money or a little, if you retain energy and enthusiasm, which cannot be bought, you can age well. Physically, emotionally, and professionally, we all have room to learn and grow. By following the simple concepts outlined in this book, you can dramatically reduce the stresses that contribute to energy drain and premature aging. I feel very strongly about honestly addressing the realities of aging, posing the questions we all have about getting older, especially to ourselves. My advice, which has turned into a mantra, is: "**Stay In Today**". I have provided many practical solutions to help you feel better with age, and I know it isn't easy. What we often take to be negative aspects of aging can be countered by *strategies to help us all feel better about getting old.*

In my career as a nutrition and fitness professional, I sought out reputable research studies that show promising results in aging well with some very simple lifestyle changes. Particularly how we can stave off the ill effects of diminishing physical capacity through improved food choices, increased physical activity, medical intervention, reducing stress, and emotional behavior change. The two things that came up over and over again were having a *positive mental attitude towards aging, and developing a community of like-minded people*, both family and friends, to keep you feeling youthful and vibrant for all your days to come. I hope these two ideas in particular help you to achieve an energetic and positive relationship to aging.

Each chapter in this book ends with a brief summary, like a book club review, which lets you go over the material presented in the chapter, and think about how to apply it in your own life. These interactive chapter summaries provide a way for you to ensure that you integrate and practice the new information you have learned, not merely read about it. You will also find a list of questions at the back of this book that provides an individual assessment of where you are right now in your life. It is not a test and you don't have to show it to anyone. They are questions that I ask myself all the time, and questions I ask others to gauge my own growth. You may find it useful to answer these questions before you start the book and again when you finish it, to see if your mindset and actions change from the beginning to the end. Once you have this information, it will help you to make better choices moving forward, and to improve your relationship to the inevitable aging process. Give yourself time and space to ponder the ideas. Some of them you may have heard a dozen times but never really considered very deeply. Others you may be encountering for the first time, and they could change your life — yes, even today!

It's one thing to read about all these new ideas and approaches — it's quite another to actually engage with the concepts and figure out to act on them so that they can help you on a day to day basis. This book is not a novel, or a biography, or a history: it is a how-to book, and only you can decide how and when you will begin to utilize the guidance provided here to help you *Eat Well, Live Well, and Age Well*. So what are you waiting for? There's no day like today to start on road! Let's all enjoy the journey together — and as the Journey song title says, "*Don't stop believin'*"!

Table of Contents

Chapter 8
Managing your Messes: Are You Oscar or Felix? 156

Chapter 9
Relationships As We Age 172

Chapter 10
Moving Forward 196

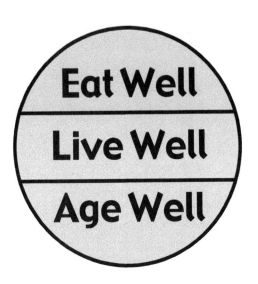

Chapter 1
Overview

Living Life to the Fullest Every Day

Our society is so youth-obsessed that we don't want to believe that one day we, too, will be old, infirm, and possibly dependent on others. Fear of aging often prevents us from living life to the fullest every day. Worrying about what might happen, hanging on to past beliefs that no longer work, and our concerns about being relevant to the younger generation can cause us to be so anxiety-ridden that we cannot enjoy where we are today. I find it very freeing to let go of old goals that are no longer realistic, release the need to seek after every popular trend, and finally just live life the way I want to for myself.

"Life Begins When you Live It, Right Now!"

Life now seems as if it is stuck on a fast-forward button. We look in the mirror and ask ourselves, "Where did the time go? How did I get to be this age? What have I done right? What have I done wrong?" At this time, there may not be answers. Don't look back on your life with regret and remorse. There is nothing you can do to go back in time. Look at old pictures of yourself and recall where you were at the time. Do you want to be stuck in the past? Don't forget that classic cliché, "Today is the first day of the rest of your life." *Life begins when you live it, right now.* This in no way means to be reckless or irresponsible. It just means to set new goals and dreams for who you are today, starting from where you really are, in the present moment. Remember my personal mantra: "**Stay in today.**"

My cousin recently said something so profound in regards to this: When driving your car, are your hands on the steering wheel and your vision focused forward on the road ahead — or are your eyes glued to the rear-view mirror (or backup camera)? This is a great analogy to the best way to navigate through life: looking forward, with an occasional glance at the past, rather than stuck in what has gone by. In fact, doing so can be downright dangerous.

"Age isn't how old you are but how old you feel" — Gabriel Garcia Marquez

The first step is to let go of the ridiculous myths and misconceptions about aging that we have all absorbed from a judgmental and youth-obsessed society — or from our own family members.

Why do people think that older people aren't cool, don't understand the youth of today, are stupid, forgetful, don't have sex appeal, and just generally are not relevant? Because that is what we heard growing up, the message is repeated in the media, and we have come to believe it. Reuters Health reports that popular music often takes negative views of aging, and the bitterness and hostility that is promoted or conveyed can be absorbed with consequences for our health — while a positive outlook can actually improve longevity. (Business Insider.com, March 25, 2016) My goal is for this book to help you reject these outdated ideas, create a new vision of healthy aging, and learn to live for you.

"Going from Invincible to Invisible"

As we age, many of us go from feeling invincible to invisible. Often we come to feel that life has passed us by. Fear and depression is common with aging. This can be a result of changes in one's own health status, or that of our loved ones. It may be an emotional response to what is going on in the world around us, or how

Negative views about aging can actually harm you: A Yale study from the Gerontological Society of America shows that negative stereotypes of aging may contribute to health problems in the elderly (Prohealth.com, July 6, 2000). Research in Psychology and Aging shows that negative views about aging can affect hearing and memory (PsychiatryAdvisor.com, December 11, 2015).

people treat us — perhaps noticing how they have begun to treat us differently than they did in the past. I have been passed over, pushed out of a line, and ignored by customer service representatives in favor of a younger person more times than I can count. You may be care-giving for infirm parents, an older spouse, or a differently abled adult child, and feeling stuck. All of these circumstances and observations can be used as opportunities to seek support, and to learn and grow.

"Older Americans are growing as a percentage of the population, and we will have increased clout in economics, purchasing power, and eventually cultural influence. If being left behind is one of your fears about aging, then starting today, be proactive in making your life the very best you can be at any age"

Let's start out by exploring what you have to offer to society as you age. I can tell you: ever-expanding wisdom, years of experience, and the opportunity to be a role model to those who thirst for guidance and understanding in a confusing world. Others need what you have to give. Older Americans are growing as a percentage of the population, and we will have increased clout in economics, purchasing power, and eventually cultural influence. If being left behind is one of your fears about aging, then starting today, be proactive in making your life the very best you can be at any age. Be active as a role model, rather than being complacent and fading off into the background. When an election cycle comes up, I often vote in favor of the older candidate. To me, their experience can be priceless!

Don't criticize young people when you sense they have shut you out based on your age. Recognize that you may have done something similar when you were young, treating your elders in a way you would not like to be treated today. Respecting the younger generations and what they have to offer you will get you further than shunning them back or criticizing their life choices.

They are the future leaders of our world. You may or may not live long enough to see their successes, but better to be remembered for your contributions than disliked for a critical and sour attitude.

"If you are a parent, take the time to teach your children, even adult children, to respect the elderly and treat them with patience, kindness and caring"

Unfortunately, many young people, from small children to young adults, have a terrible attitude towards the aging. If you are a parent, take the time to teach your children, even adult children, to respect the elderly and treat them with patience, kindness and caring. Over and over again, I have seen how parents and other adults can contribute to this lack of respect that the youth have towards older people. I will be sitting in a restaurant and hear an entire family making fun of other patrons who are overweight, old, or just don't look or act the way they think they "should." I have also seen crowds of teenagers, often accompanied by their parents, pile into an elevator, and leave an elderly or wheelchair bound person sitting there, left behind, ignored, and often stunned and ashamed. This may be part of a harsh society of bullying those who are "different" — but we should realize that at some point, we will all be old. Take advantage of the opportunity to model and teach compassion, acceptance, tolerance, empathy — we will all benefit from it eventually. I remind my teenage daughter and her friends to be aware of how they treat older people, especially their parents and grandparents. I always think of the meaningful song, "*Teach Your Children Well*," by Crosby, Stills and Nash.

Act Your Age

As noted in the introduction, I came very close to making this the book title. Rather than the admonishment we remember from childhood — **Act your age!** we were scolded if we were acting childish — today it is a reminder to embody the fullness of the lives that we have lived, and not pretend to be younger than we are. In my mind, it is a reminder to live your best life at the age you are now. Participate in life doing the things that you want to do and truly enjoy, rather than doing what you are told you are supposed to like, or acting as if we really enjoy every hot new trend.

The quest for eternal youth is pervasive across North America, and it is making its way around the globe. In business and in social settings, it seems we have lost all respect for the elderly, and what they have to offer to society. We turn away from images of the elderly, and shun them in social settings. Yes, people over 50

> The older population grew from 3 million in 1900 to 46 million in 2014. The "oldest old" (those 85 and over) grew from just over 100,000 in 1900 to 6 million in 2014 — and is projected to grow to 20 million by 2060, possibly even sooner as death rates at older ages continue to decline (Older Americans 2016: Key Indicators of Well Being)

are showing up more in movies, television, and magazines, but we still have a long way to go. The advertising industry targets a demographic that is so young, they are ignoring the fact that in America, we have 70+ million people over 50 years old, a whole new set of demographics for the population that is over 60, 70, 80 and beyond. This huge market segment can be catered to with new products and services that can be provided for us, by us.

Your peers are your best advisors. When you surround yourself with your contemporaries you will see how far you have come. While you may gain energy and insight into current trends by hanging around people who are 10 or 20 years younger, it can also put you at a disadvantage, worrying that you don't fit in, and that they may feel the same way about you. This discomfort can be relieved upon finding a social network of people that you can relate to, where you can find that unspoken common ground that we all need. I put tremendous effort into spending time with my four siblings (we are very close in age), as well as with my childhood, high school and college friends.

"When you use your age-related experience and surround yourself with like-minded and similarly-aged people, you will flourish"

It is very important to surround yourself with people who make you feel good about who you are. Sometimes it's just an unspoken awareness that you have people that you can be yourself around, versus people who can make you feel horrible with just a look. Be with those who make it easy for you to "act your age" and not feel like you have to try to be someone you're not — at least, not anymore. Aim to cultivate friendships with people who have a positive view of aging. You don't want to surround yourself with people who are depressed or critical about aging themselves, that can bring you down even more. Positive perceptions of aging include viewing the later years as a time of continued growth and learning, when relationships are developed and maintained, and feelings of control over the aging process lead to health behaviors such as good food choices, regular physical activity, making new friends, and enjoying social support, greater life satisfaction, and increased longevity (Mather Lifeways, Institute on Aging).

Life Is Short, Even When You Live To A Very Old Age

Life moves at warp speed, and you will be beamed up before you know it. Every moment counts, and by slowing down to realize that, you will feel that the days are longer and more full than you

> Eat well tip: Seek nutrition from food or vitamin supplements to improve mood and attitude. Make sure you get enough calcium, chromium, folate, iron, magnesium, omega-3s, Vit. B-6, Vit. B-12, Vit. D, and Zinc. Being physically active also lifts your mental outlook.

ever imagined. You can never get your time back, and you won't forget the past, but learn from it. If you stay stuck in your "should-have-done, could-have-done," life will pass you by. Most of us are just good people who want to continue to enjoy our lives, be healthy, live long, and age well. Doing all the things we like, that make us happy and feel complete is a common goal. Looking at the issues facing us as we age helps us cope with these issues, work through them, and feel fulfilled.

"Life moves at warp speed, and you will be beamed up before you know it"

Life seems to move faster for two reasons: one reason is that each year is objectively a smaller fraction of your life when you are 50 than when you are 5. That is why it seemed like an eternity to get to your next birthday or holiday when you were a small child, while they are on an onrushing treadmill today. The other reason that time seems to move faster as we age is that we get into routines and habits that require little thinking or awareness, which leads to the sensation of time passing quickly. (CareerSidekick.com, March 3, 2016) The key to slowing down the pace is to seek out new and unusual experiences in order to create memories that stand out. Zimbardo and Boyd, authors of *The Time Paradox*, recommend focusing on positive (vs. negative) past memories, living in the present, and "envisioning a future full of hope and optimism." (PsychologyToday.com, April 5, 2010) *Focus on the present, try new things, and have a positive outlook on the future, in order to create memories and slow down the perception of the passage of time.*

"Just remember, when you're over the hill, you begin to pick up speed" — Charles Schultz

One of the best ways to live life to the fullest and enjoy each day is to stop comparing yourself to anyone else, whether it's a friend, a family member, or especially someone you have never met, much less a photo in a magazine! Celebrities and other extremely wealthy people in the public eye don't seem to age the way we mere mortals do. You never know what tricks they use to look good on the outside. Why focus on someone else's life? It is wasted energy.

"Aging is not lost youth but a new stage of opportunity and strength" — Betty Friedan

Either you are now, or hopefully, one day, you will be old — but we all dread becoming that elderly person that no one seems to care about. One way to combat depression about getting older is to be grateful that you are aging; it is wonderful to have a long life, see changes in the world, and know your children, grandchildren, and extended family and friends throughout life's most profound milestones.

Older adults understand the value of technological changes more, because they can appreciate what it took to get to where we are today, and what life was like before these new inventions existed and were part of our daily lives. We may remember asking our parents about what life was like before television — our children ask us about what life was like before cell phones or the internet — we can only imagine what our grandchildren will be asking about.

"Ask an older person about their lives, and share information about your own with someone younger, to encourage communication and respect between generations"

When we, the baby boomers, were little, the world was enormous, and now it seems smaller as time goes by. I always loved to hear stories from my grandparents and parents about what the world was like before I was born. Certainly, nothing can stop the passage of time, but rather than see it fly by and feel we have achieved nothing of note, let us make the connections that make living worthwhile.

One step you can take today is to *find a person older than yourself and ask him or her to share something from the past*, or some knowledge about an area of interest. I am certain that you will be very surprised at what you can learn. I love interviewing people I meet on my travels about their world travel tips — they provide great insight and practical information about where to go and how to best organize my trips. Then pass along the favor, and find a young person who is interested in what you have to share, and tell them something about the world before they were born, or offer information you have that would be of value to them today.

"Do not grow old, no matter how long you live. Never cease to stand like curious children before the great mystery into which we were born" — Albert Einstein

All of this is humbling and ennobling at the same time, and it provides living examples of the value of older people, their experience and knowledge, and why they are worthy of respect rather than disdain. It's so enlightening to see the world through someone else's eyes, and know that life will go on after they are gone.

How and Why We Age

Contrary to widespread belief, while "good genes" can be a plus, "bad genes" do not account for all of what ails us. Scientific studies show that less than 25% of longevity can be attributed to our genes. (Journal of Gerontology, March 27, 2012) As we age, genetic inheritance becomes less of a factor and environment and lifestyle become more important.

"Scientific studies show that less than 25% of longevity can be attributed to our genes" (Journal of Gerontology, March 27, 2012)

From the time I was a child, I was told that my life would follow the same path as my parents and grandparents. My family would always tell me, "No matter what you do, you will be fat, all the women in our family are as they age." I was also led to believe that I was stupid and wouldn't amount to much because I struggled in school, and was too afraid to ask for help. When I decided to maximize my potential, despite my "bad genes" and meek demeanor, I really fought back. I took on a wellness lifestyle in my early 20s that I have kept up over the years, and it has shown me that genetics are really just a small part of the equation: I have seen and shown that choices about how well you live affect how well you age. Keep in mind that the older we get, as we surpass the diseases and infirmities that were predicted for us, genetics becomes less of a factor and environment and lifestyle become more and more important.

> **"We can enhance our mental, physical, and emotional capabilities as we grow older by continuing to learn, be active, reduce stress, and remain involved with our friends, family, and community in a positive way"**

How we live has the most profound impact on our health as we age. Behaviors such as not smoking, making healthy food choices, enjoying regular physical activity, adopting a positive attitude, and focusing on mental engagement with life are not inherited — except insofar as we copy the examples set by family members. In short, we are responsible in large part for the quality of our own old age. We can enhance our mental, physical, and emotional capabilities as we grow older by continuing to learn, be active, reduce stress, and remain involved with our friends, family, and community in a positive way.

There is a mistaken belief that older adults, with age, have a dramatic decline in physical and mental capability. This assumption finds its most pronounced expression in the general belief that sexual

Eat well tip: You don't have to eat the same foods you grew up with, or that the rest of your family eats. You can choose to keep flavors and seasonings, changing food preparation methods and swapping some ingredients for more healthful options.

interest later in life is rare and downright inappropriate, despite demand for HRT (Hormone Replacement Therapy) for women, and Viagra for men, which shows that sexual activity is alive and well among older people.

> **"I have made a rule about such things, which I commend to you... As soon as you feel too old to do a thing, do it" — Margaret Deland**

Decades of research debunk the myth that to be old is to be sick and frail. Throughout the world, older people are generally healthy, only a fraction being part of the "elderly infirm." Even in advanced old age, the majority of the elderly population has little functional disability, and the proportion that is disabled is being whittled away over time. There is increasing momentum toward the emergence of a physically and cognitively fit, nondisabled, active elderly population.

The combination of longer life and less illness is adding life to years as well as years to life. We will examine a number of ways to enhance our lives by improving our food choices, expanding our physical activity, increasing our social circles, and uplifting our mental and emotional outlook.

> **"Old age has its pleasures, which, though different, are not less than the pleasures of youth" — W. Somerset Maugham**

Blue Zones

National Geographic partnered with longevity expert Dan Buettner, author of a fascinating series of books about "Blue Zones," studying the world's longest-lived people to discover their secrets to longevity. They noted that while the average life expectancy for Americans is 78.2 years, over 70,000 Americans reached the ripe old age of 100 this year. What can we learn from those who live the longest, and is it possible to "reverse engineer" the reasons for their longevity?

The five areas — or "Blue Zones" — where people had the highest proportions of people who reach age 100 include the Barbagia region of Sardinia (world's highest concentration of male centenarians); Ikaria, Greece (lowest rate of middle age mortality and lowest rate of dementia); Nicoya Peninsula, Costa Rica (lowest rate of middle age mortality, second highest concentration of male centenarians); Seventh Day Adventists in Loma Linda, California (who live 10 years longer than other North Americans); and Okinawa, Japan (females over 70 are the longest-lived group in the world).

What do the residents of these varied and far-flung areas have in common? A team of medical researchers, anthropologists, demographers and epidemiologists found nine evidence-based common denominators they all shared:

Move Naturally. Nope, you don't have to work out in the gym or train for a marathon, just live in a way that makes you move constantly without thinking about it. Grow a garden, build a treehouse, walk up and down stairs, and don't rely on modern appliances to reduce your house and yard work activities.

Feeling of Purpose. Having a reason to get up in the morning can add up to seven years of life expectancy. In Japanese this essential feeling of motivation is called "Ikigai," in Spanish "plan de vida" — what is it called in your life?

Reduce Stress. Even people in these heavenly Blue Zones experience stress, caused by work worries, family concerns, financial pressures, health issues. Stress can lead to chronic inflammation, which is linked to most age-related diseases. What these longest-lived people have are regular ways to reduce stress: Okinawans remember their ancestors, Adventists pray, Ikarians take a nap, Sardinians have happy hour. Find your own route to reduce the negative impacts of stress.

> **Eat well tip:** Try these Blue Zones approaches to eating: Stop eating when you are 80% full; eat smaller meals later in the day; add more veggies, and reduce your intake of animal products, perhaps enjoying 1–2 meals per week where you eat vegetarian.

Follow the 80% Rule. stop eating when you are 80% full! The 20% gap between not being hungry and feeling full could be the difference between losing weight or gaining it. And remember the saying: "breakfast like a king, lunch like a prince, dinner like a pauper." The late afternoon or early evening is the time when Blue Zone folk have their smallest meal, and then they don't eat again until they break their fast in the morning. Natural intermittent fasting helps to keep them trim and guards against illness.

Focus on Veggies. Beans of all types are the protein source at the center of most meal plans followed by centenarians. Many of them eat meat only about five times per month, in small serving sizes, 3-4 oz., about the size of a deck of playing cards, and the vegetarian Adventists shun animal products altogether.

Wine is Fine. Except for the teetotaling Adventists, all the other Blue Zone residents drink moderately and regularly — just 1-2 glasses per day, with friends and/or with food, preferably a local wine. Do not save up all week and binge on the weekend with 7-14 drinks, there is no benefit in being drunk.

Community. Nearly all of the centenarians interviewed by National Geographic belonged to a faith-based community. Research shows that attending religious services regularly can add 4-14 years of life expectancy. The social support aspects of belonging to such groups are notable.

Family First. Blue Zone families are extended families, with aging parents and grandparents nearby or in the home, which lowers disease and mortality rates for the children in the home as well. Being in a committed relationship, and investing in children with time and love also reaps rewards: up to 3 years of life expectancy for being married, and children who will be more likely to care for you when it is needed.

Healthy Society. If you're not lucky enough to be raised in a family that values healthy behaviors, you can choose one for yourself. Okinawans create *"moais"* — groups of five friends who commit to each other for life. Studies show that smoking, obesity, physical activities, happiness, and even loneliness are contagious. Choose your social networks with health in mind, and select those that will encourage and support your own healthy choices. Join a gym, a local running club, or an online nutritional support group.

While genetic makeup will certainly help you get to 100, most of us can make it well into our 90s without chronic disease. By adopting various aspects of a Blue Zones lifestyle, we can increase our average life expectancy by 10-12 years. (Dan Buettner, Reverse Engineering Longevity, November 2016)

Fear of Aging and its Implications

Often, it seems as though our society is obsessed with the negative rather than the positive aspects of aging. There are widespread misconceptions that older people are a frail, powerless, sexless, and ugly segment of our population. Just look at all the youth, beauty, and sexual enhancement products dominating the media! They are all focused on younger people, and ignore the values of older adults. This can generate fear in us that we're becoming irrelevant, and are being discarded by society, or at least by younger people.

"Don't Fear Your Face — Face Your Fears!"

It is very helpful for our personal growth to understand how we are perceived by others around us. While we may imagine that their views are overwhelmingly negative, it's probably not as bad as you think. Worrying about how others see us tends to come in waves: some days we may feel that everyone around us is looking down on us or judging us harshly; on other days we may recognize that they respect our experience, history, accomplishments, and outlook — or maybe even our sassy fashion sense, positive frame of mind, fitness routine, or our health and well-being — despite our advancing years.

"What I have found is that I only feel better about myself if I am working on my self-esteem, rather than my appearance"

Personally, I have struggled with this a lot. I do a lot of public speaking and I often wonder if I fit the image I am trying to portray, of eating well, living well, and aging well. There is a trend towards doing extreme makeovers, facelifts, dangerous diets, and wardrobe overhauls that cost a fortune. I have tried facial injections to tame my frown lines, I dye my hair to cover the grays, and use expensive facial care products. *What I have found is that I only feel better about myself if I am working on my self-esteem, rather than my appearance.*

We all know that some days are better than others, based on our current mood. Some embrace aging as a blessing, and work hard to make the most out of their time — while others may become bitter, hostile, resentful, and really difficult to be around. A positive attitude will help you engage in life for years to come, and make it easier for others to enjoy your company. Indeed, older folks with a sunny outlook tend to draw people to them, happy to be around someone who sets an example for how to *Eat Well, Live Well, Age Well.*

"You don't stop laughing when you grow old, you grow old when you stop laughing" — George Bernard Shaw

By this point, you know what you like, how you like to dress, what you like to eat, and so on. You're no longer trying to keep up with every fashion trend whether or not it works for you, or aiming to impress others by visiting the latest hot restaurant or nightclub or vacation spot. Stick to what works for you and have a relaxing third act rather than go along with someone else's plans for you.

At the same time, keep an open mind and continue to learn and grow, try new things, and explore ideas and places that are new to you. This can help you to remain flexible and feel relevant. Adapt your likes and dislikes to feed your personal growth, rather than hardening into a shell based on explorations and decisions made years — or even decades — earlier. You may find that new fitness, food, and fashion choices may energize you in ways you never anticipated, and help you to face aging with a more positive frame of mind.

Just Say No

Say "no" to demands that no longer work for you. Learning to take care of yourself is not selfish, it is essential for your survival. This is particularly important if you have others in your home that you are taking care of, too. Looking after children, aging parents, or maybe an infirm spouse, wears everyone out. It is astounding how resourceful my daughter and husband become when I have had enough and take a little time off from caring for them!

Genuine Fears About Aging

Most fears about aging are related to self-care: loss of independence — including being unable to drive — declining health, running out of money, death of loved ones, isolation, and fear of falling or hurting oneself. (Caregiverstress.com, March 2, 2011)

Some fears are related to performance or appearance, slowing down and losing one's edge, suffering from painful joints or difficulty walking or enjoying activities, creeping (or sudden!)

TAKE TIME FOR YOU

Plan self-care into your schedule, the same way you do a work meeting or doctor's appointment. Spend the time and budget for a massage, a visit to a spa or sauna, a healing walk or vigorous hike in nature, swimming or boating or whatever you like to do. Enjoy reading a book, leafing through a magazine, watching a serious drama or light-hearted TV show. Keep a date with yourself for daily physical activity, healthful food preparation, a trip to a museum or the movies. Make time for your favorite craft activities such as sewing, quilting, needlepoint, embroidery, carpentry, collage, scrapbooking and more.

Write the appointment into your calendar, and don't arrange anything that will interfere with this time for yourself. It is as important for your health and longevity to reduce stress and improve your outlook, as it is to visit your health care professional or take your medication. This is for you and you alone, so whatever it is you need, take it. Even if it is as little as five minutes alone, or luxuriating in a bubble bath for two hours, it is up to you and you deserve it.

weight gain, sagging skin, wrinkles, grey hair — and the sense that it is inevitable, unavoidable, and too late to do anything about our bodies or our health. (Joan Pagano, Beliefnet, 2017)

Some of us experience professional fears, related to anxieties about younger associates at work taking your place — as well as not recognizing yourself in the mirror, loss of lucidity, and fear of death. (Gail Saltz, Health, March 8, 2017)

All of these fears can be addressed, and it is never too late to begin to make positive changes that will result in improved outcomes.

"Eating well, regular physical activity, community engagement, and reducing stress to live a quality life will improve your chances of aging well, and being a happy senior citizen"

Everyone wants to be as happy and productive as possible for as long as possible. While some centenarians, mostly from the Blue Zones discussed above, seem to age without paying attention to what they did to achieve that milestone, most of us need to be conscious of what we do in order to enjoy life past 70 or 80 years of age. Eating well, regular physical activity, community engagement, and reducing stress to live a quality life will improve your chances of aging well, and being a happy senior citizen.

"I have chosen to be happy. It's good for my health" — Voltaire

As noted above, scientific evidence shows us that lifestyle plays a larger role in how we age than our genetic makeup. America is soon going to have a good portion of our population over age 60, a highly productive generation that will most likely be able to contribute to society well into their 80s and 90s. One of the many bestselling books by Olympic runner Jeff Galloway is entitled *Running Until You're 100*. (When asked about this book, Jeff jokingly replies, "After 100, you're on your own.") Jeff himself is in his 70s, and runs a marathon every month, along with his wife Barb. Fewer than 1% of people run a single marathon in their entire lives, much less one every 30 days. The Galloways, and others like them, are redefining what we think of as the "oldest old" and how they live on a day to day basis.

Much of this is due to a huge reduction in life-threatening illnesses in the twentieth century, and people being more proactive about their own healthcare. Precursors to chronic disease such as high blood pressure, high cholesterol levels, and smoking are declining in the elderly now, because now it is cool to be healthy at any age. Cultural impacts are important: haven't you noticed how the "cool" characters in old movies all smoked — and today, only the "bad guys" do? Reducing smoking, obesity, stress, and increasing activity can all help us to achieve greater longevity and a happier, healthier life.

"Planning ahead helps you to feel in control of the aging process: plan meals, workouts, savings program, living arrangements, and your fears will lessen as you take charge"

A great way to reduce fears about aging is being as prepared as possible for whatever may come your way — financially, physically, nutritionally, medically, emotionally, mentally. Planning is everything. You have heard the expression that "Luck is what happens when preparation meets opportunity." Sound planning and hard work are needed to help you meet and greet the challenges of aging with a positive attitude.

I didn't take this seriously because I always thought I had a cushion with my birth family and then with my husband. As we experienced financial ups and downs, and lost loved ones, I really started to worry about my future and planning for old age. Now that I have handle on this, I feel a lot less stress about it. This book is here to be your guide as you plan out what you want to do to achieve the quality of life and longevity you seek.

Taking Risks

Risk taking can have many benefits, but the pros and cons need to be constantly evaluated to see if the risk is worth a potentially favorable outcome. If you are one of those people who are 50 or older, but think and often act as if you are 25, pay close attention to this information.

You can manage your risks in life by taking the following steps: consider the anticipated good time or need to take a risk against the possible consequences. For younger people who tend to feel immortal, this includes the use of drugs and alcohol, indiscriminate sex, driving without a seatbelt, stealing, lying, gambling, and adventurous stunts including extreme sports such as free climbing and cave diving.

On one hand, these activities can make you feel carefree and youthful; on the other hand, the consequences can be dire, especially as we age and we don't bounce back quite the same way that we used to when we were younger. Many of us think of the Steppenwolf song title, "*Born to be Wild*," and conjure up images of Peter Fonda in *Easy Rider*, coolest guy ever! But rather than go bungee jumping or spelunking or cave diving... how about you start out small, and safer!

> ## "Don't try to be young. Just open your mind. Stay interested in stuff. There are so many things I won't live long enough to find out about, but I'm still curious about them" — Betty White

I was always terrified of heights and that phobia prohibited me from doing many things I would have liked to experience. I finally got up the courage to go zip lining in the rainforest of Costa Rica. I was safely hooked up on the harness and did a few runs from 200 feet to 1000 feet. It was fabulous, and when I was done I felt I could do anything! This is what successful risk-taking will do for you. Be careful and be wise.

For older people, this all needs to be considered, in addition to recognizing your diminished ability to heal from accidents, threats to your livelihood, reputation, and jeopardizing your family's health and safety. Even small risks may not be worth it; why walk balancing on the edge of a narrow wall, when a fall could result in serious injury and resulting lifestyle change?

Ask yourself a few basic questions before taking these kinds of risks:

Does the risky behavior fit with your basic values and goals?

Are you lonely and looking for a way to fit in with a crowd?

Eat Well, Live Well, Age Well

Are you trying to prove — to yourself or someone else — that you're just as tough, strong, brave as when you were younger?

Are you trying to show off, or surpass someone you're angry with?

On a positive note, taking risks can translate into fulfilling your potential. While it may be seen as "risky" to train for a marathon, a triathlon, a surfing event, a masters body building competition, or a senior tennis match, if you follow a proven training plan you can achieve unimagined results within your capacity. This can inspire not only yourself, but others around you to achieve new goals and improve their health and longevity. Just keep in mind that health is the priority — not "winning" — so take better care of yourself every day, and choose your risks wisely, with the goal of improving your well-being, rather than overtaxing your system.

Interactive Chapter Review

Living Life to the Fullest Every Day. *Society is youth-obsessed. Are you? How does this affect your opinion of yourself? Your spouse? Your friends? Younger colleagues? Your children?*

What concerns do you have about aging? Are you worried about your health, your finances, becoming irrelevant at work? What old goals can you release that are no longer serving you? What new goals can you create that would feed who you are today? How can you let go of any regrets for roads not taken — or figure out how to take them at last?

What myths and misconceptions do YOU have about aging? Do you show any of those in your own life? How can you combat these wrong ideas in society?

Are there specific challenges you are facing that makes aging difficult? Physical health issues of yours or a loved one? Problems at work, issues with friends or family members? Are you in a caregiver role? How can you use these as opportunities for growth?

What expertise can you offer to the younger generation? Can you sew on a button, balance a checkbook, edit a sentence, build a bookcase, plant a garden, manage a team? Who can you help with your wisdom and experience who would be grateful for such assistance?

And what do you have to learn from younger people in your circle? Are there aspects of technology, physical fitness, travel, or food planning that you could learn about? How about new phone apps, new exercise approaches, new ways to travel, new nutrition information? Just as you like to be listened to and have your ideas and opinions respected, young people do, too — you can give them a caring and attentive ear.

How can you model and teach young people in your circle to have good attitudes towards the elderly or people with different physical abilities and appearances?

Act Your Age. *What does it mean for you to "act your age?" What are you doing that is perhaps inappropriate for you, that you would like to let go?*

How can you demonstrate respect for your age peers and seniors, at work and in your community? Do you have a business or marketing idea that could serve this huge and growing demographic?

While you may understand new trends by hanging out with younger people, you will have more comfort in a network of people you can relate to and who have similar experiences to yourself. How can you create or deepen such a circle of friends in your own life?

Life is Short, Even When You Live to a Very Old Age. *"Life moves at warp speed, and you will be beamed up before you know it."*

Every moment counts, what can you slow down to appreciate in your life today? What "could-haves" and "should-haves" can you finally let go of, so you feel that your life is full and rich, just as it is?

Can you name people in your life to whom you have compared yourself, either with superiority or jealousy? Cousins, friends, high school classmates, colleagues? How about celebrities, or people in the news? Do you say, "I wish I had that life" when you read about the rich and famous, or "thank goodness I don't have that life" when you hear stories of those who struggle with poverty and disease?

How free would you feel if you stopped comparing yourself to these people? Would you be more able to focus on your own goals and desires?

The world has changed a lot in our lifetimes — and more in the lives of those who are older than we are. Ask older folks about their lives, and take the time to share your own experience with a younger person. Think of someone you can do this with, right now!

How and Why We Age. Genes are not everything; environment and lifestyle are more important as we age. Have you "given up" changing things that are within your control, using the excuse that "everyone in my family is X" (i.e., fat, sedentary, diabetic, has heart failure, etc.) What can you do now to improve the quality of your life?

Do you still smoke? Drink to excess? Make poor food choices? Resist or avoid regular physical activity? Harbor negative opinions and hostile views towards the world and the people around you? Are you willing to make changes in any of these areas if it will improve the quality of your life?

Do you believe that older people have a dramatic decline in physical and mental capacity, and lose their interest in sex? Or do you believe the research that shows older people are generally healthy, and becoming more so? If you feel that "going downhill" is inevitable, what can you change in your day to day activities, that will help you to add life to years as well as years to life?

Are you able to say "no" to things that get in the way of your taking care of yourself? Do you schedule your self-care appointments first, and keep them as seriously as a work meeting or doctor's appointment? What kind of self-care do you enjoy most: Gym workouts or long runs? Meal planning and prep? Spa treatments like massage, facial, sauna? Cultural dates with yourself at a museum, movie, or just reading a book? Craft projects such as sewing, quilting, carpentry? Outdoor walks or hikes?

Blue Zones: 9 Common Denominators. Five "Blue Zones" where people often live to be 100: Sardinia, Ikaria Greece, Costa Rica, Seventh Day Adventists, Okinawans — what do they have in common?

1) Move Naturally (be active on a regular basis)

2) Feeling of Purpose (know your "why")

3) Reduce Stress (daily rituals)

4) Follow the 80% Rule (stop eating when 80% full)

5) Focus on Veggies (increase vegetable intake, reduce or eliminate animal products)

6) Wine is Fine (in moderation)

7) Community (regular services)

8) Family First (live with/close to aging parents and grandparents)

9) Healthy Society (form or join a group focused on healthy choices)

While genes can help, adopting a Blue Zones lifestyle can increase life expectancy. Which of these 9 areas do you practice now? Which would be the easiest for you to adopt or improve? Which would be the hardest to incorporate into your life?

Fear of Aging and Its Implications. What common misconceptions do you see about aging in the society? How do they make you feel?

How do you think others see you? On your bad days? And on your good days?

Are you generally angry and bitter, or do you manage to keep a positive attitude? What could help you to reduce the former and increase the latter?

Are there favorite styles or activities that you enjoy and that work for you, regardless of whether they're in fashion or not? What are they? Or are you still trying to keep up with the latest trends? How does that work for you?

Are you stuck in a rut, reluctant or afraid to try new things? What could help you to be more flexible and open-minded?

What lifestyle choices have you made in the past that may have reduced your longevity? Which ones could you change now to increase your lifespan?

How do you see yourself continuing to be an active, productive, contributing member of society into your 60s, 70s, 80s, 90s? What plans can you make today to help you achieve these goals?

Taking Risks. *Are you a risk-taker or risk-avoider? Do you tend to go out on a limb, and if so, why? Are you trying to prove you've "still got it"? If you're a risk-avoider, what could help you to challenge yourself safely to achieve new goals?*

Can you change your focus and priority from "winning" or "facing danger" (or avoiding risk) to "improving health and longevity" in order to reach new heights safely?

Chapter 2
Life Begins When You Live It

Be Here Now

Life begins when you start to live it, right now, today. As you are now. You can start anew at any age, but you must begin where you are, in reality. Then every step you take moves you forward, moves you upward, towards actual achievement and change. There's no value in regretting the past, or that you're not further along than where you actually are. Accept and embrace yourself as you are.

I have vivid memories of being a teenager and listening to the song, "We've Only Just Begun," by the Carpenters. Wishing and hoping my life would turn out perfect, and the man of my dreams would sing Frankie Valli songs to me. Neither one happened, but I turned out okay, and I can deal with anything I don't like about my life today.

In this chapter, I address topics that are very heavy and require deep thought and self-examination. If you are having a difficult time with your emotions, I suggest reaching out to a close friend or relative that you can trust and ask them for an hour of their time to just listen to you without judgment. Offer to listen to them in return and you will both feel better afterwards. This is something I often do with people near and dear to me. It is very helpful and will save a lot of money in therapy bills!

The reasons behind this concept are no mystery. It is behind most spiritual teachings to "be here now," to be mindful and aware of the present moment. The past is gone, and the future is not promised to us — all we have is today. And the present, for those of us moving forward in years, is very good indeed. By the time you reach 40, hopefully you've already made most of life's biggest mistakes — maybe more than once.

You have been around long enough to differentiate a con job from someone who's legitimate. You can tell a trustworthy person from a flake. You've been in the work world long enough to know what you're talking about, and your expertise counts. You're probably finally starting to earn some real money, and you're mature

Explore the web to discover sites that explore and extoll the benefits of turning 40: Lifehack.org gives us 8 things you learn by turning 40: Age is just a mindset, confidence, wild and crazy days are over, goodbye to drama, don't change yourself to be liked, "no" is a complete sentence, be comfortable in your own skin, and the best years are ahead of you.

Also from Lifehack.org, 20 life lessons we learn by age 40 including: find what you love and own it, don't fear mistakes, you deserve respect, romance is not the same as love, you win some, you lose some, not everyone is always going to like you, money is not the measure of success, the past has passed for a reason, so let it go, and so on.

enough to recognize the value of saving and investing rather than going on a spending spree (although you do enjoy the pleasures in life). Most importantly, even if you are down to a handful of close people in your circle, you know who your real friends are, and you can surround yourself with a strong support system.

By 50, hopefully you have reached the point where you can rely on your instincts to get by. The truth is, you have had that ability your whole life, now you need to trust it! You can feel when there's a genuine connection with someone, whether you've just met them or if you've known them for years. You recognize the value of giving back, and investing time in your long term relationships. You know when someone is lying, you know when someone is giving you the cold shoulder, and you know when someone is trying to manipulate you or take advantage of you.

Address these things head on, because you can. Life is too short to let others screw things up for you. If old friendships become abusive, and you no longer find pleasure in the other person's company, feel free to draw back and develop new connections with others who feed who you are today. In the workplace, don't be afraid to be the whistleblower, or at the very least speak out. It is better than the constant abuse and resentful feelings that go along with staying silent.

Try this approach: when you walk into a room and there are people throwing the proverbial "daggers" at you, hold your head up and remember they are doing it because you have something they want. Aloofness will get them every time!

> **"The great thing about getting older is that you don't lose all the other ages you've been." – Madeleine L'Engle**

Celebrate Your Life

One wonderful way to celebrate your life is to have a party on your birthday. I am amazed at how many people are embarrassed of their age, and think that cake, candles, cards, gifts, and singing "Happy Birthday" are just for kids. This seems to get ingrained in the psyche at an early age. You are never too old to have a party, and unlike the usual holidays that fall throughout the year, this is yours and yours alone, a day you don't have to share with anyone.

Many people have bad memories of birthday celebrations gone wrong, or perhaps your birthday is associated with a personal or national tragedy. Some just don't like acknowledging publicly that they are actually a year older. My mother in law claimed to be 39-plus when I first met her, and she was still 39-plus at her 100th birthday party! Starting this year you can change that, and erase any negative connotations that irk you every year. You have earned the right to celebrate another year of life!

I love my birthday. I have had bad ones and good ones. In the past, every milestone birthday was a huge disappointment for me because I thought that every 10 years I would have accomplished everything I set out to do for that decade. Of course, I always fell short! But despite my personal anxiety, and even at my lowest point when I had suffered many personal setbacks and losses in a given year, I never stopped celebrating my birthday, and being grateful for the gift of life that comes with it.

"The longer I live the more beautiful life becomes." – Frank Lloyd Wright

Another thing that can make a birthday fun is a keepsake, photo or scrapbook from your special day. Take a picture on your birthday and jot down a few thoughts about where you were at the time, how you felt, what job you have. This is a great way to have a chronological history of your life. Keep a record of the lessons you learn, the wisdom you gain, and the values you hold and reflect upon them.

> **Eat well tip: It's your birthday, enjoy your birthday cake! If you can't or won't have cake, have fresh fruit, sparkling water or even a non–food celebration such as a dance party or walk in the park. Just enjoy the company of others, and celebrate your life.**

If you have old pictures lying around, put them in albums. Even if they are not in chronological order, they will be preserved for years to come. Don't worry if you haven't done this in past years: life begins now, when you start to live it! Start this year, and enjoy it as a new tradition going forward.

My daughter and I have started doing this for family celebrations, and it's a wonderful bonding experience. If your photos are all on your phone, download them and create a virtual scrapbook, with pictures and your own notes to remember how you felt on that day, who was there, how you were feeling, etc. This is not only good for your own memories in the future, it is a beautiful legacy for your family.

Goal Setting and Goal Getting

It is good to have weekly, monthly, and yearly goals, even at an advanced age. Goals should be clear, practical, and measurable. Time goes by so quickly, 3, 5, 10 years from now you can be still

Daily Goals: Start every day with some specific goals in mind. Just taking a few minutes to write down a list, or to run the items by a friend or family member, is really helpful. Also, it helps on those days when you feel like "I got nothing done" to check the list and see that you actually did quite a lot!

At night, before bed, take note of what you accomplished. Don't worry about what you did or didn't do, just start to pay attention to how you deal with it and what changes you would like to make going forward.

Many people find it valuable to read a daily meditation book or other guide first thing in the morning to provide a framework for their day. These often include an inspirational story, a quote, or a thought for the day, which you can focus on when you're feeling distracted.

Or you may prefer a practical tracking guide, such as an exercise journal in which you list your activity, the weather, how you felt while participating, which sneakers you wore, etc. — or a food app where you track meals, water intake, calories, or macronutrients such as carbs, protein, and fat. Whether it is handwritten or online, these often provide structure and guidance to help you progress towards larger goals.

checking accomplishments off your bucket list! Always plan time for relaxation, trips, family, and hobbies. Advancing careers, repairing damaged relationships, being grateful, spending time with friends, volunteering, and earning more money, are all good things to strive for, things that will make you happy and relaxed as the years go by.

"Growing old isn't so bad when you consider the alternative." – Anonymous

There are so many opportunities to accomplish goals in ways you may never have imagined. If I am not feeling accomplished or creative, I just think about one thing I would like to get done that day. It is eye opening to write down your day and see how much you actually did do, or how you can better plan your day to see your efforts come to fruition.

Emotions As We Age

Living with regret is a common problem that starts even in early adulthood. We all look back and realize how much time we have wasted worrying, especially about things we cannot change. This wreaks havoc on our self-esteem and our ability to move forward. As you get to a more advanced age, you will look back and see the futility in that.

The proverbial "Mid-Life Crisis" hits most of us at a certain age, where we have things about ourselves that we like, things we don't like, things we can change (whether we choose to or not), and then the realization that it is too late for some things to change, and you need to make the best of it!

"Turning 50 — At this stage of life, winning or losing no longer plays a role. Just the effort and completion of a goal alone will be enough to you to feel a tremendous sense of accomplishment"

The things we cannot change are the most painful to examine. Did you wish you had pursued that job? That romantic interest?

Fought back the wrongs that were done to you or your loved ones? Well, now is the time to put the past aside, and realize that everything that happened before today is a done deal. If you spend any time on it, you are wasting today's precious moments.

Let go, let loose, let yourself be free. This doesn't mean to be reckless or careless, rather to be adventurous. You don't even have to travel abroad to learn about a new country. Take a book about some foreign land, sit in the backyard, and get lost for an afternoon. Expand your brain by studying a new language with one of the free online programs.

You aren't going to qualify for the Olympics at this stage of the game, so enjoy the challenge of trying out a new sport for fun. I took up long distance running at 34, and have completed many marathons and half-marathons well into my 50s. At this stage of life, winning and losing no longer plays a role. Just the effort and completion of a goal alone will be enough to you to feel a tremendous sense of accomplishment.

Although you never know — look at Sister Marion Irvine, the "flying nun": Having been sedentary and a smoker, she took up marathon running NEAR AGE 50, and in 1984 was the then-oldest person to qualify at the Olympic trials at age 54! She went on to break numerous age-group records, including the world record in the marathon for female runners over 50 with 2:51:01, and continuing to break age-group records among 55-59 and 60-62 year old female runners.

> ## "Age is an issue of mind over matter. If you don't mind, it doesn't matter." – Mark Twain

Most of us, of course, will never achieve these kind of results, and will simply have to benefit from the wonderful side-effects of being an adult-onset runner, such as low blood pressure, reduced aches and pains, increased mobility, improved sleep, happier mood, and so on! Thinking about this always reminds me of the song title, "Young at Heart," because we'd all like to feel like that.

The Impact of Stress

One of the biggest obstacles that keep us from achieving wellness is stress. Anxiety, panic, uncertainty about the future, loss of loved ones, the unknowns in life, are among the many stressors that are beyond our control. Emotional and physical stress can cause anxiety, sleeplessness, and inability to concentrate. Unexplainable aches and pains emerge. Uncontrolled stress can also lead to an early death, because it wreaks havoc on our immune system.

Life will always have stressors, but how we manage them is key. Aging in itself can cause chronic stress. Illness, job instability, loss of family members, and children and parents living far apart from each other can cause a real sense of insecurity. Chronic stress, where the body remains in a perpetual state of high alert, also known as fight or flight response, prevents the body from calming down, and as a consequence you never feel fully rested, and yet you are always tired. Think of this state as a constant adrenaline rush.

Cortisol, known as the "stress hormone," is released in response to adrenaline to protect the body from short-term threats. The immediate effect is to keep the body and the mind sharp by raising the heart rate, blood pressure, and blood sugar. It also diverts blood from the digestive system to the bloodstream and enhances muscles to help us work quicker and more efficiently. Cortisol will almost instantly lessen our awareness of pain, and heighten all of the senses, including memory.

The downside is the longer your body's cortisol levels are elevated, the more wear and tear on the body's endocrine system. You are more likely to accumulate excess weight and producing more visceral fat, and then cardiovascular disease and metabolic syndromes, like type 2 diabetes, can kick in. Prolonged high stress situations can suppress the immune response, making it harder to fight off germs and infections. It is then more likely that you will get sick. Our brains are also adversely affected, because long term stress can also cause a decline in cognitive function.

This is the true meaning of "burnout." You cannot always articulate how this makes you feel, but you know you are too wiped out to function and make sound decisions, and yet you don't have a solution.

> **"You gain strength, courage, and confidence by every experience in which you really stop to look fear in the face." – Eleanor Roosevelt**

My Experience With Stress

I have always been "High Strung". My response to stress was always overreaction and being ridden with fear. I tried every form of stress reduction techniques out there and yet nothing was working. I developed unreasonable phobias that inhibited me from enjoying many things and it stunted my emotional growth. I eat really well, exercise every day, and go out of my way to make friends, yet I always felt wound up, worried, and stressed out.

When I gathered up the courage to take a good hard look at the way I live, I found some changes I could make. Number one was reducing the caffeine and sugar in my diet. I always minimized the effect it had on me because coffee consumption and lots of it was part of my culture. I started drinking coffee in my teens and it was a ritual among my family and friends to drink it all day long. A few years ago I started to drink half decaf and then reduced the number of cups I was having in a day. Then I went to all decaf and eliminated any other food products that contained caffeine and refined sugars. I save sugar for those rare occasions like my birthday or a family milestone to have a bite of cake. It is remarkable how much better I feel and how much easier it is for me to handle stress. The other life changing habit I embraced was sleeping more. I am no longer worried what anyone thinks if I leave a party early to go to bed, take a nap in the afternoon, or sleep late on days where my schedule is flexible.

Everyone is different, but perhaps some of my other changes would help. Try adding more natural foods and reducing additives and prepared foods, becoming more active, and focusing on improving relationships with those closest to you. Lastly, don't be afraid to consult with a doctor if your high stress continues despite positive lifestyle changes. Medical professionals may offer other insights or solutions that you haven't thought of yet, and that could help you.

"As much as you may not be at fault, your response to stress will dictate how happy you will be. Take an inventory of what is important and worth your time, and focus on what you can control"

The Benefits of Exercise in Stress Reduction

Exercise at any level will counter the extreme fatigue we feel when stress is overwhelming. Any movement is known to produce energy and the positive hormones that make you feel good. Instead of viewing a workout as yet another chore to cram into an overstuffed and overcommitted day, we can see it as an opportunity to improve our mood and attitude, and thus be able to cope better with all of our other obligations.

One of the advantages of exercising in the morning is that it can lower your body's cortisol levels for the rest of the day. This will help you manage the entire day in a more relaxed fashion. When the body is calm, you can think clearly and open yourself to new thoughts and ideas. But beware of over-exercising, as that can also cause an increase in cortisol. Balance is critical.

"Exercise and application produce order in our affairs, health of body, cheerfulness of mind, and these make us precious to our friends" – Thomas Jefferson

As much as you may not be at fault, your response to stress will dictate how happy you will be. Take an inventory of what is important and worth your time, and focus on what you can control. Life will be a lot more relaxing. You may not be able to control the circumstances and events in your life, but you can begin to take control of how you respond to them.

Study the nutrition and fitness chapters in this book closely. Many people have found that improved dietary habits, including vitamin supplementation and increased protein consumption, can improve mental outlook. And physical activity, especially cardiovascular workouts that cause increased blood flow throughout the system and to the brain, has been shown to reduce stress hormones, resulting in improved sleep patterns and a more positive attitude in general — aside from the obvious health improvements that come along with a healthy diet and active lifestyle.

Who knows which comes first: depression, anxiety, and stress — or eating poorly and not taking care of oneself? Did something

Eat well tip

Aside from exercise, food choices can affect your cortisol levels. Seek out foods that are as close to nature as possible, so your body doesn't have the stress of dealing with "frankenfoods" filled with chemicals and additives that need to be screened and eliminated. Certain foods help to lower cortisol, including magnesium- and zinc-rich foods, microgreens, Omega-3 fatty acids, and citrus fruits. Provide a balanced diet and supplement as needed to ensure you are getting all of the nutrients your body requires to live well and age well.

Certain vitamins and supplements have been shown to reduce cortisol levels, including Vitamin C, B vitamins, and Zinc. In addition to these, others may help improve mood and may reduce stress and improve sleep, such as Vitamin A, Vitamin D, Calcium, St. John's Wort, Melatonin, Kava Kava, and Valerian Root. You may wish to try adding these to your daily routine to see if they help you to feel better and perform at your best.

Journal of Compliments and List of Gratitudes

One unusual approach to improving your mood and self-esteem is to start the habit of writing down five compliments about yourself every day. As with the theme of this chapter, these compliments must be based in reality. Rather than other journaling practices you may have tried over the years, of examining your flaws or areas which need improvement, this practice is simply to write down five positive things about yourself. They may be very simple: for instance, if you cleaned the kitchen that day, you might write "neat and tidy." Or if you were productive at work, "hard working." If you prepared lunch for your children, "thoughtful." If you took time to visit a sick friend, "kind." If you work out or go for a long walk, "fit and active." If you make good food choices, "health conscious."

Continue this practice for several months — or years — and you will have a long list, and a handy reservoir of positive thoughts about yourself: you are dedicated, loving, supportive, organized, thrifty, capable, talented, a good parent, helpful, considerate, healthy. What a much better inner voice to hear than the usual carping and self-criticism!

For "advanced" work you can add three things for which you are grateful that day: health, life, children, family, work, home, and so on. Gratitude lists are more commonplace than lists of compliments, but both practices can help to improve your mood and outlook — as well as your own self-concept — especially when continued on a daily basis for a period of months. It's amazing how quickly these can have an effect on your daily life.

happen in your life that made you sad or lose interest, causing you to eat "comfort foods" and lie around the house? Or did you start relaxing your dietary habits and exercise regimes, which led to feelings of lethargy and general malaise? Rather than analyze it, just address it head on and make the change!

> **"Men do not quit playing because they grow old — they grow old because they quit playing" - Oliver Wendell Holmes**

Add more energizing foods to your day, such as vegetables and lean proteins and healthy fats — incorporate movement throughout the day, walking farther, perhaps trying out a new and challenging activity such as Zumba, belly dancing, surfing, or rock climbing — read books about nutrition and sports physiology, and you'll begin to see the positive effects in your own life, day by day.

Coming Clean and Clearing Your Conscience

I am convinced that one of the reasons for premature aging, or difficult aging, is holding on to emotions, especially ones due to fear. You will be astounded at how clearing the conscience of harbored emotions will make you feel alive and vibrant again.

One way to free yourself of negative emotions is to pay back your debts. They can be emotional or monetary, but should be resolved. Walking around with a financial debt hanging over your head is probably one of the most stressful places to be, especially if you owe money to friends or family. If you cannot pay back the whole debt, offer to pay a portion, an ongoing percentage, or offer a trade or barter to settle the matter at last. The offer alone will lift the heaviness that comes with the shame of not having the ability to pay it off.

Continuing to avoid this situation will also keep you feeling poor and financially undernourished. Taking steps to address and hopefully resolve these issues will give you a new lease on life, the freedom to be and do what you want, and hopefully the support of those who have helped you in the past, as they see you working to make good.

Learning from the 12 Steps of Recovery

Many people have found freedom from alcoholism, drug addiction, overeating, codependency, and other issues through following the 12 steps. If God is not your thing, turning it over to a higher power of your choice will still work. If you or a loved one is suffering from these issues, seeking out one of these support groups can lead to a major life change for the better.

1. We admitted that we were powerless and that our lives had become unmanageable.

2. Came to believe that a Power greater than ourselves could restore us to sanity.

3. Made a decision to turn our will and our lives over to the care of God as we understood God.

4. Made a searching and fearless moral inventory of ourselves.

5. Admitted to God, to ourselves, and to another human being the exact nature of our wrongs.

6. Were entirely ready to have God remove all these defects of character.

7. Humbly asked God to remove our shortcomings

8. Made a list of all persons we had harmed, and became willing to make amends to them all.

9. Made direct amends to such people wherever possible, except when to do so would injure them or others.

10. Continued to take personal inventory and when we were wrong promptly admitted it.

11. Sought through prayer and meditation to improve our conscious contact with God as we understood God, praying only for knowledge of God's will for us and the power to carry that out.

12. Having had a spiritual awakening as a result of these steps, we tried to carry this message to others, and to practice these principles in all our affairs.

If you owe someone an apology, call him or her and do it. Apologizing when necessary frees you up in ways you cannot imagine. If that is out of your reach or impossible due to death or incapacitation, write it down to help let it go — or do a charitable deed instead! If someone owes you an apology, don't throw it in his or her face, either you get the apology or you don't. Maybe the other person doesn't even know you feel you deserve one.

I had a situation with someone who I was very close to, who became angry at me for not being there for her as much as she was for me. I was going through a very bad time in my life and needed so much support, I didn't realize how self-absorbed I had become due to my pain. When she confronted me, I apologized, and thankfully she accepted it. What it taught me was that my unhappiness made me behave in a selfish manner, and I didn't even realize it. If someone is seeking an apology from you, take a look and see if you did in fact play a role in whatever made this person angry at you — even if you had a good reason for behaving the way you did, it's good to take responsibility for how your actions impacted the other person.

When Others Have Hurt Us

For those of us who have a situation where we suffered a terrible wrong at someone else's hands, it can be very difficult to let this bitterness and resentment go. After all, they deserve it! How can we forgive genuinely destructive or negative behavior by others?

The best way to do this is to realize that holding on to negative emotions only hurts us, not the other person. We're the one with the anxiety, the heartburn, the lack of trust, the mysterious backache or headache, the depression, the emotional pain. By letting this pain and bitterness go, it doesn't mean we forgive or even forget the bad behavior or injury done by the other person: it just means that we are no longer responsible for punishing them in our minds and in our hearts on a continual basis for what they did to us in the past. It is time to move on, and feel the freedom and happiness we had before this injury every occurred, perhaps with a bit more wisdom to avoid such an event in the future if possible.

People from different faith-based systems have various approaches to letting go of resentment against those who have done them

Whatever path you take to improving your health, start by eliminating the people, places, and things that get in your way and that you don't need anymore. Let them go with gratitude for all they have brought to your life, and with hope they will benefit someone else — or at least, they won't clutter up your personal space anymore.

Now is the time to gently rid yourself of people who no longer serve your best interests in your life. If you are entangled with someone who is a family member or part of a social circle that makes it awkward, step away slowly. Spend less time engaging with them and more time away. See how it makes you feel. If it has a calming effect on you to stay away, then pay attention. Sometimes it is just bad chemistry between people and that can bring out the worst behavior in all of us. Your exit will not only benefit you, but will defuse the situation and make it easier on everyone involved.

I have done this myself, bit by bit reducing the time I spend with someone who is difficult or makes me feel uncomfortable, and while it may be challenging at first, in the long run everyone feels better.

wrong, including praying for the person who has caused them harm, turning the other cheek, or rather than wishing them ill to wish them every benefit they want for themselves. Sometimes studying these different paths can provide some solace or guidance on how to deal with anger and resentment in your life. Perhaps you can write a letter to the person who hurt you, and put down all of your pain on paper. That may allow you to release it from having to carry it around in your head and your heart all the time, casting a shadow over every moment.

I found for myself when I feel that someone has hurt me or done something terrible to me — and its happened more times than I care to remember, a lover, a friend, a work colleague — I now go to a place of compassion. If people are treating you unkindly, taking advantage to you, being mean or dismissive, you may be wishing them harm and feel vengeful. I can assure you that their lives are probably miserable already, and must be in shambles emotionally. You don't need to add to that, just be thankful for your own happiness.

> **"Nothing is inherently and invincibly young except spirit. And spirit can enter a human being perhaps better in the quiet of old age and dwell there more undisturbed than in the turmoil of adventure." – George Santayana**

It is never easy to move on from a truly painful situation, even one that occurred years or decades earlier, but the effort is worth it right now. If you have carried this pain with you for a long time, it may even be hard to get rid of it, since your identity may have become entwined with the pain. Worse still, trying to dull or hide the pain may lead you to other unhealthy behaviors, such as drinking too much, using prescribed medication inappropriately or resorting to illegal drugs — or even by escaping from your feelings through overeating, excessive exercise, or extreme religiosity (yes, there can be too much of a good thing).

If you can find a way to let go of past wrongs, you will find that you have a new opportunity to discover yourself, free of bitterness and resentment, right now, today. Again, don't regret the years that you suffered — surely you have learned from that experience as well, and can share that with others to help them let go perhaps sooner than you were able to do so.

I told you this was going to be a challenging chapter.

Dealing With Emotions As We Age

Your health and happiness should always come first. It is not at all selfish to reduce or eliminate people, places, and things from your life that are distressing and counterproductive to your well-being.

Even when it comes to family members, you have a right to put a stop to behaviors that jeopardize your health, wealth, and physical and emotional wellness. All of the emotions we deal with can be handled in a positive way to make your life better.

> **"Your health and happiness should always come first. It is not at all selfish to reduce or eliminate people, places, and things from your life that are distressing and counterproductive to your well-being"**

Anger is a necessary emotion. I know I get angry sometimes, but I know that's okay. We are often told that it is futile to be angry. You have a right to it and you should embrace it, but always remember to direct the anger outward at the perpetrator or situation, not yourself; anger turned inward becomes depression. Harboring anger in the form of resentment hurts you more than the one it is intended for; getting angry at someone is no more effective than getting drunk at someone — the only person who gets hurt is you. Unresolved anger says more about your inability to forgive than what the other person said or did, no matter how unforgiveable it may have been. Expressing anger verbally is much preferable to acting it out in violence that may harm others, or suppressing it in ways that may harm yourself.

> **"I have learned now that while those who speak about one's miseries usually hurt, those who keep silence hurt more." - C. S. Lewis**

Vengeance is carrying around an extreme form of resentment that results in looking for ways to get back at people who have harmed you. Whether it is personal or business, people have a way of mastering the art of it, scheming, planning for the kill, and it almost always never happens. Vengeance should have no place in your life. It is especially self-destructive to harbor feelings of vengeance towards people who are no longer in your life. People have hurt you because they are selfish and seeking their own benefit, or are insensitive and don't care about you (or anyone

---

else), or they simply don't know any better. The more time you spend dwelling on the wrongs that were done to you in the past, the less you have for yourself and to create positive memories for the future. Keep in mind that somewhere along the line, you may have hurt someone else and didn't know or didn't intend to. Would you want that person walking around hating you for the rest of his or her life?

Envy is an involuntary, visceral response when someone has what you want, and you think or know you cannot have it. The best way to defuse this is to acknowledge your feelings and try to stay calm. Even when warranted, envy makes you do things that you will regret because you don't think clearly when you are comparing yourself to another person's success and failures. You never know what another person's struggles are, where they came from, or where their personal choices will lead them. Wishing harm on another can bring it back to you in ways you least expect, and may not always be pleasant. Your strengths and weaknesses, accomplishments and failures, will always dictate your current mood, and your ability to make sound decisions.

Jealousy is a form of possessiveness, in which you have fear that someone else may take something that is yours, whether it is your spouse, your child, your work, your money, etc. Jealousy can often lead to hostility, fights, violence and over-protectiveness, attempting to defend what is "yours" against others you think are trying to take it from you. Have faith that your loved ones stay with you because of your own value, and would not run off at the slightest invitation.

"Be not afraid of life. Believe that life is worth living, and your belief will help create the fact." – William James.

If you are in pain, whether emotional or physical, its common to either retreat or attack. Fears, past experience, and your own instinctive reaction, all contribute to your current response. Take a deep breath, count to ten, think before you act — all of these approaches can help to quell a sudden reaction or rash action that you may regret later. Take a good look at your current belief system, whether it is based on your upbringing, religion, or habits and feelings you discovered later in life, and see if it all still works for you, and helps you to cope with unexpected or negative responses to difficult situations you may encounter.

Often, we can develop a very high threshold for unacceptable behavior from ourselves and others because it is what protected us when we were young and fighting our way through the world. If you have said to yourself, "I'll let him/her get away with it this time, but never again," and yet it keeps happening, you now need to look at yourself. As we age, this can be so frightening, but it is time to put an end to accepting bad behavior from those who are in your life. We want to be open to new people, new experiences, and continue to learn and grow; this is impossible if we have to close down our emotions in order to tolerate really intolerable actions from others. Being closed and defensive is very alienating, especially later in life when we really need supportive people around us.

Don't Judge A Human By Its Epidermis!

Whatever you do, do not judge a human by its epidermis! Your perception of the world around you and the people you meet will dictate all of your choices, good and bad. Everyone loves to consider him or herself a great judge of character, but we also base our assessment of someone on a first glance. However, remember that what you see on the outside is not always indicative of where a person is at in his or her life. Your outlook may be marred by past hurts — sometimes a word, a look, the way someone is dressed, will form an impression on you that is negative. You may be so needy for others to accept you that will let anyone into your life. I have been on both sides of this terrible catch-22, and it took a lot of internal work to reach a point where I became discerning as to who I would let into my life. You never know what someone has been through, or where they are going. Unless you feel that you or your family is in immediate danger, it is better to step back, let the person prove himself worthy, rather than make a snap judgment that might be detrimental to all involved.

"Every human being has value and should be recognized for all of his or her accomplishments. Any contribution small or large should be celebrated"

Many of us were abused as children, both physically and emotionally, which may have not been acknowledged at the time. In prior generations, for many parents there was a fine line between appropriate discipline and abuse, and behavior that today would be shunned was then widely accepted. Now we all know the repercussions of this philosophy of parenting. As a result, many of us have severe issues with self-esteem that led to making decisions that were not in our best interest. Consequently, we repeat these behaviors because it feels natural to us, and we don't know how to change it.

Start by acknowledging that your current behaviors are often a response to old feelings and learned patterns of behavior, and as dysfunctional as they may be, it's your comfort zone. You'll be surprised once you verbalize what you are really thinking and feeling, and share what you think are your secrets, how very

Statistics on child abuse and neglect are startling, with over 3.6 million reports each year involving almost 6 million children, including 45 children who are killed each day. Consequences and risk factors on those who survive are wide-ranging, but include repeating the pattern, as well as suffering from other disorders and mental illnesses as a result. (americanspcc.org/child-abuse-statistics/)

freeing it all is, and how many others have similar experiences. It may feel so hard to get started, but you will find it is well worth the effort.

Owning Your Life

In order to become your true self, you must face the reality of where you are today in every aspect of your life. The myth in our head, that when I am rich, fit, married, single, retired, my life will be better....... We always imagine that we will be happy if we lose 20 pounds, get that raise, can hold that yoga pose, move to a bigger (or smaller) home, the kids go to college, we retire, etc.

"Happiness is an inside job"

But the truth is, happiness is an inside job. None of these external changes or achievements can "make us happy." As Abraham Lincoln once famously said, "Most folks are about as happy as they make up their minds to be." Your expectations of what life should be like will dictate how well you handle what is thrown at you. Life is never going to be completely the way you want it, not even most of the time.

"Old age ain't no place for sissies." – Bette Davis

When you are able to be honest with yourself, and to be honest about what's going on in your life, you can really be your authentic self. When we start to accept our life just the way it is now, embrace feeling lost, scared, overwhelmed, weak, whatever it is that we may be feeling, we can start to make changes for the better. But we have to start from where we actually are, right now, not from where we imagine or wish we were.

The key is to start somewhere. Forget the "all or nothing" mentality and celebrate the small improvements that make life better for you and those around you. Try doing something for someone with no expectation of return or recompense of any kind, a true charitable act. Pay for someone behind you in line at the grocery, or put money in someone else's meter — and don't tell anyone about it. Contribute time at a soup kitchen or homeless shelter.

Do good deeds for their own sake, not for external recognition, or hopes that your friends or children or spouse may one day return the favor.

And especially if you're someone who is always doing for others: learn how to ask for help yourself. Take a practice run with a family member, a friend, or neighbor to see how it feels to let someone do something for you without any strings attached. You would be surprised at how much it improves your well-being, while giving you the reality check you need to engage in the world as a real person. You don't have to be a superhero and do everything yourself. When you show someone else who you really are, you will accept who you really are. The more often you do this, accept being comfortable with the here and now, the easier it becomes to be just in today.

I don't think anyone is 100% happy and content all the time. It's okay to be sad, depressed, melancholy, remorseful, wistful, and even angry sometimes, but it is not healthy to hang on to it. Feel your feelings, but don't let them move in and take over your life.

There are also situations in our lives that are really not acceptable and it is important that you address them, for your own sake. When you are in the depths of a situation that is not in your best interest — and remember that is not meant to be selfish, but to maintain your self-preservation — you should take action. If you are feeling resentful, stuck, and worst of all hopeless, it would be helpful for you to find an outlet, and a permanent solution to alleviate your distress. Whether it stems from a stressful work environment, family problems, or social situations that you feel you cannot confront, try to find a way to mold a life that finds you some peace and happiness.

I am always telling people to eat well, exercise, and find ways to reduce stress. If you have physical and monetary limitations, the nutrition and fitness chapters contain information about ways to achieve wellness at many levels of capability. When coping with hardship, whatever that may be, take ownership of your life. Know that if you are the healthiest you can be, you will be more able to face whatever hardships life is throwing at you.

This is a better solution than the seemingly easier route, of turning to drugs or addictive behaviors — even the legal ones, including alcohol or out-of-control relationship with food and even fitness — to try and cope. Everyone struggles at some point in their lives, and for some it is worse or more prolonged than others. If you are completely honest with yourself, you will find that what you are struggling with now is mostly likely a re-occurring theme in your life. The good news is that it will show you that the struggle is always there, but it doesn't have to dictate your happiness.

When you experience pain, whether it be physical or emotional, it is very real. It doesn't matter if the person next door has it worse, or you have obligations that prevent you from addressing what is going on in your life, your pain is yours and it is real. Share your thoughts with a close friend or family member and get some feedback on how you seem to others. More often than not, you will find that it is normal and everyone goes through it.

If your pain doesn't begin to diminish through your own efforts, you may need professional help, and reaching out would be very good. As noted above, there are recovery programs for every

Eat well tip

Rather than turn to typical "comfort foods" to help you cope with a difficult situations, think of healthful, energizing foods that will actually provide to nutrition to improve your life. Raw foods and live foods often give us connection to the earth. Sometimes just a glass of fresh, clean cool water is enough to turn around a sad mood and lift us out of a funk — you might not be depressed, just dehydrated! Don't make a bad situation worse by slathering it with ice cream, cake, candy, fast foods, or alcohol. Take control of your food choices, even in difficult circumstances, and you will see your situation improve.

ailment that plagues our society. Seek out a support group that speaks to you, and you will find how much it helps not to feel alone in your struggle. Learning from others who have been down the same road, and are coping with the same issues, can provide guidance when a way out seems impossible. Consulting with experienced and compassionate medical, psychological, and spiritual providers may also offer support beyond what you can get from family or friends or self-help groups.

As we age, we realize that there is no "getting there," no perfect place or way to be. Our childhood fantasies of happily ever after, and achieving a perfect life, never seem to make it to fruition. We often feel after giving it our all, the reward should be a stress-free, problem-free, easy life. It is unproductive to keep hoping for a life that will never be fully at peace. The feelings of failure following this are pervasive, but if you can see hope, and have the courage to pursue change, your life will get better at any age.

The tiniest effort, a small change, can make a huge impact on your happiness going forward. Just make up your mind to be as happy as you can be, and you'll find yourself well along the road to being there. The one thing that I think is ageless is happiness. It is never too late to find something to smile about.

Interactive Chapter Review

Be here now. Life begins when you start to live it, right now, today. Accept and embrace yourself as you are.

Have you already made most of life's biggest mistakes? What were they? What did you learn from them?

What have you achieved in your life thus far? Are you more mature, more financially stable or savvy?

Can you rely on your instincts more than you did when you were younger? How do you do this?

What is the value of giving back and investing in old friendships? How do you recognize people's character?

Are there relationships that no longer serve you? Can you reduce or sever the amount of contact with this person?

Will this make room to welcome new, more positive people into your inner circle?

How do you celebrate your birthday? Are there any negative associations with the day or date you want to change going forward? Can you release any anxiety about not meeting certain goals by a particular age? Have you started a birthday scrapbook, real or virtual? Do you have any alternate ways to celebrate your birthday?

Goal Setting and Goal Getting. Do you have weekly, monthly, yearly goals? Goals should be clear, practical, and measurable. What are they?

Do you suffer from regrets? About what? Does this affect your self-esteem? Have you experienced some kind of "mid-life crisis"? How did it manifest itself?

What will help you to put the past aside, enjoy the present, and set new goals for the future?

What new things will you try? Pick up a new sport or other activity? Learn a new language?

The Impact of Stress. Does stress have an impact in your life? Do you suffer from physical symptoms, aches and pains, illness, that are stress related?

What do you do to help relieve stress? Can you improve your food choices, increase your physical activity, practice positive journaling?

What stressors do you have in your life today? Do you care for children, parents, family members with disabilities? Do you have issues at your job, or have you suffered traumatic losses? What do you do to help manage your stress? Have you found that regular exercise can help to moderate anxiety, depression, and burnout?

Try the Journal of Compliments and List of Gratitudes, based on real things that you do every day, and real things in your life you value. See what effect this has on your self-esteem over several months.

Do you have personal debt? Can you start to repay it and clear your books? Even beginning to address it will relieve some tension.

Do you owe someone an apology? Can you make it in person, or write it down for someone who is no longer here? What about doing a charitable deed instead, what could you do instead of an apology?

Emotions As We Age. *Are you harboring bitterness or resentment over something someone else has done to you in the past? Can you figure out a way to let it go? Realize that holding onto these negative emotions causes you pain but does nothing to the other person.*

It is never easy to let go of this kind of pain, especially if you've had it for a long time. Rather than suffer regret, perhaps you can help someone else by sharing your experience of holding onto these feelings for too long.

Putting your own happiness first is not selfish. Put a stop to behavior by others that damages your heath, wealth, physical and emotional wellness.

Anger may be a necessary emotion, but resentment is not. Anger turned inward becomes depression. Unresolved anger says more about you than the other person, no matter what they did. If you dwell in resentment, you may begin to form feelings or plans for vengeance, which should have no place in your life. Envy and jealousy can also cause emotional pain.

If you are in pain, emotional or physical, do you retreat or attack? Can you slow down your instinctive reaction and take time to think before you act, so you don't do something you regret? Think of an instance where you acted too quickly and made a situation worse.

Is there any unacceptable behavior by others in your life? What can you do to reduce or minimize its effect on you? Do you have to walk away? How else can you keep yourself open and able to trust?

Judging Others. *Do you find you jump to conclusions when meeting people based on their appearance? What they wear, their weight, skin color, age, religion, politics, where they live, what kind of car they drive, what they do for a living, if they're married or single? Can you step back and let them show you who they are before you make a judgment?*

Did you experience abuse or neglect as a child, even though it may have seemed "normal" at the time? Has this had an impact on your self-image as an adult? Did it make you accept behavior from others that was actually detrimental to you? What can you do to change this built-in response?

Owning Your Life. *Do you maintain a myth that "things will be better when I...." or "I will be happy when I...." (fill in the blank)? What will help you to realize that happiness is an inside job? What can you do to help you decide to be more happy? Can you donate some time to charitable endeavors? Can you ask someone to help you with something?*

Are there situations in your life that are unacceptable, at work, in your family, in social situations? What actions can you take to maintain your self-preservation?

Can you improve your nutrition and increase your physical activity to help reduce your stress levels? This can help you cope with whatever hardships life is throwing at you, more so than turning to drugs or addictive behaviors.

Can you identify patterns in your life, where you are struggling with the same issues, perhaps in different forms, throughout your life? Once you recognize it, that may help you to address it once and for all. Talk to a friend or family member about what is causing you pain, or seek out a self-help support group or professional advice.

What can give you courage to keep going and pursue change, once you realize that "happy ever after" is just for fairy tales?

Chapter 3
The Physiology of Aging

How and Why We Age

The secret to aging well, commonly referred to as successful aging, is to enjoy every minute of it. Contrary to widespread belief, having good genes is a plus, but doesn't account for all of what saves us from an early demise. As we age, genetic inheritance becomes less of a factor and environment and lifestyle become more important. How we live and where we live begin to have a more profound impact on our overall health.

> ### "As we age, genetic inheritance becomes less of a factor and environment and lifestyle become more important"

It is a myth that to be old means you will be sick and frail. Today, most people in their 50s, 60s, and 70s are generally healthy. Even in advanced old age, the overwhelming majority of the elderly population is functioning very well. There is an increasing trend toward the emergence of a physically and cognitively fit, non-disabled, active elderly population. The combination of longer life and less illness is adding life to years as well as years to life. We see more and more highly active adults nowadays participating in life in ways we never thought possible. There is a trend of elderly adults between 50 and 70 attending college, taking up surfing or skiing or skydiving in their 80s and 90s, and even 100 year old sprinters and marathon runners!

> ### "Since 1900, average U.S. life expectancy has risen from 47 to 79 years of age"

With advancing age, there is the reality of a natural decline in the efficiency of the cardiovascular system, as well as a slowing metabolism. We tend to decrease our activity which exacerbates this decline, along with a weakening of the immune system, which inhibits the body's ability to stave off disease. The less we exercise and watch our food intake, the more pronounced this becomes.

Another contributing factor, known as the Telomere theory, is the concept that all of our body's cells have a life span. As the chromosomes within cells replicate, the telomeres (the DNA sequence at the end of their "legs") get shorter and shorter. Telomere shortening has been linked to many aging-related diseases, and once telomeres become too short, cells are unable to divide ("replicative senescence") and the body eventually stops living. Oxidative stress, free radicals, and obesity have been shown to shorten telomeres, while antioxidants and caloric restrictions may preserve them. There are so many products on the market today that claim to reverse aging on a cellular level, but buyer beware! If these products really work as well as they appear, we would all stay 21 forever.

Your time here on earth may be predetermined, or may be the luck of the draw, but your choices in life will dictate how well you live as you age. Such behaviors as eating a healthy diet, getting plenty of exercise, not smoking, moderate alcohol consumption, and the ability to engage socially, are not inherited. In short, we are responsible in large part for making it to the golden years, and enjoying ourselves once we get here. By following a plan to enhance our mental and physical capabilities as we grow older, we will find that life is so much more fulfilling that we feared.

Three Key Functions of Aging

There are three key functions of aging that everyone worries about:

Your Brain

Just about everyone experiences some memory loss as we age. This doesn't mean that you can't function, it just is a sign that we need to start paying closer attention to our actions. How many times have you looked for your glasses, just to find them on your head, or worse, you are already wearing them? Key chains have a life of their own. You think you put them in the same place every day but yet you keep losing them. You have to look at the keypad on your phone to remember a number.

Now you know why your grandparents and parents seemed to be acting crazy when you asked them to do something simple. It just gets harder as you age. It can be very helpful to make lists and paste them near your telephone or on the refrigerator, put your keys near the door, and reduce the clutter in your home and office. Does it help to eat blueberries and take gingko biloba and do crossword puzzles? Maybe, but organization is key to staying sane as you age.

Your Eyes

Right around age 40, your eyes weaken more rapidly than they did before. I'll never forget the fateful day when I could no longer see the exit sign at the end of the office hallway. I turned to my friend and said, "I must be tired." She said," No, you need glasses!" She lent me hers, and I had a moment of clarity, both physically and mentally, that stuck with me for good. Contrary to popular belief, if you ignore the signs of aging, life isn't as much fun.

One option to correct your vision is Lasix surgery. This is a procedure where the doctor puts cuts in your retina to correct your eyesight. If you are concerned about having the surgery, you may want to start with a great pair of fashionable glasses, or try contact lenses. Whichever way you decide to go, don't squint, it is bad for your eyes and causes wrinkles. If you cannot see, you may end up avoiding or snubbing your family and friends because you don't recognize them — and worst of all, you will miss out on the successes of your loved ones because you couldn't see them celebrating milestones throughout their lives.

Your Skin

You wake up and keep seeing this tired person in the mirror. At first you think, "I didn't get enough sleep. I should have gone to bed earlier. My kids are too much to handle. My work is too demanding. My spouse doesn't help out enough." But then, even after a vacation, a good facial, lots of makeup, you still look tired and those lines seem to be permanent. You run out and buy expensive creams that promise to reduce fine lines, and stave off wrinkles... to no avail. The reality sinks in: you have wrinkles.

"Contrary to popular belief, if you ignore the signs of aging, life isn't as much fun"

You become obsessed with skin care regimens. Some of us consider invasive procedures such as injections or surgery to try to turn back the hands of time. In fact, more than just some of us — Americans spent over $16.5 billion on cosmetic plastic surgery in 2018. You ask all of your friends and family, "Do I look old?" You imagine that no one wants you anymore, and you are too old and uncool to fit in anywhere. We'll talk later about how to deal with these feelings!

"Wrinkles should merely indicate where smiles have been." – Mark Twain

You can minimize this natural process with good skin care, minimum exposure to the sun's harmful rays, and finding ways to reduce your stress and improve your rest. To protect your skin from sun damage and cancer, use sunscreen liberally with an SPF of at least 15 when you walk out the door, up to SPF 30 whenever you spend any time outdoors. Reapply regularly, and avoid direct tanning, including the indoor tanning booths. Excessive UV exposure also raises the likelihood of developing skin cancer (more on that later). Get a consultation from a dermatologist for a skin care regimen that is right for you, and easy to follow. Keep your bathroom counter uncluttered: surprisingly, the more beauty products you buy, the less you will use them.

"Wouldn't you rather have laugh lines than frown lines?"

I notice a big difference in my skin when I get sufficient sleep. I am nocturnal and tend to be at my best late at night. This isn't compatible with the way the world works, so as long as I have to get up with the sun, I make an effort to get in bed 7-8 hours before I need to rise. Even if I lay in bed in read, it results in more rest than if I am up late wandering around the house or watching television — and my skin definitely benefits from this "beauty sleep."

The best thing you can do for your skin is be happy. Finding the things in life that make you smile really helps reduce the ill effects of aging, relaxes the body overall, and makes you more receptive and open to new experiences. Wouldn't you rather have laugh lines than frown lines?

"Old age is like everything else. To make a success of it, you've got to start young" - Theodore Roosevelt

Examining the Aging Process Through the Decades

In Your 20s

The 20s are time when we are usually finishing our education, and are expected to be responsible, but don't really know how. Growing up, graduate school, working on your career, getting married, starting a family is emphasized in these years, but these goals are often antagonistic to what most 20-somethings want, which is perpetual freedom. Society has made us worry so much about our future, that young people seek more and more outlets to relieve stress. Many of these behaviors have harmful consequences, such as drinking and drug use, stress eating, reckless promiscuity, being irresponsible in the workplace, and becoming estranged from family.

The effects of aging are seen in the skin as early as the 20s, when fibers that keep skin taut begin to weaken. Eating well and exercising are critical starting in early adulthood, because the average American gains between 0.4 and 1.8 pounds per year through middle age. Fertility for women begins to decline in the late 20's, so while having children before age 30 may be a challenge with all of the other interests for those in their 20s, it might be the only opportunity for many.

In Your 30s

Everything you have done up to age 30 sets the tone for later in life. Even though turning 30 can be a trauma for some, most people still feel vital and invincible. For some, the hair starts turning gray because hair follicles stop producing the pigment melanin, and by

35, two in five men are showing signs of male-pattern baldness. Skin becomes dry, and lines start to form.

Bone mass begins to break down faster than new bone forms, and gradually we begin to lose muscle mass. Even if your weight remains constant in your 30s, there is atrophy in muscle tissue and an increase in body fat. Metabolism starts to slow down, fertility drops, and the juggling act of balancing family and work leave a lot of people in this age group sleep deprived and haggard. Diabetes, whether due to hereditary factors or lifestyle choices, starts to show up as early as age 30. Luckily you can still bounce back by eating well, exercising, and getting sufficient sleep.

> **"At age 20, we worry about what others think of us. At age 40, we don't care what they think of us. At age 60, we discover they haven't been thinking of us at all." – Ann Landers**

In Your 40s

As you approach 40, your appearance starts to change. Skin cells divide more slowly, causing the skin to thin. You start to see the beginnings of age on your face, wrinkles form around the eyes and mouth, and is a little harder to keep your weight in check. Starting at age 45, cancer becomes one of the top causes of death, and the risk of heart disease goes up for men. The lens of the eye is gradually growing stiffer, a condition known as presbyopia, a type of farsightedness. Sounds gradually grow more muffled and high frequencies may drop off as eardrums begin to lose elasticity.

The cruel irony of turning 40 is that you feel like you have seen it all, heard it all, and you start to not care what others think. It is a time when we should feel optimally confident, and yet the outside world starts to look at you differently. Over the hill, past your peak, etc. On the plus side, your career is established, and your earning power peaks. There is such a wide range of lifestyles among the 40-somethings. While some couples in their 40s are having babies, others are becoming grandparents. Some have already lost their parents, while others will have theirs for another 20 to 30 years.

Some are juggling child-rearing and caring for aging parents simultaneously.

The 40s also begin a decline in the hormones that have dictated so many aspects of sexual behavior and identity since puberty, both for men and women. As estrogen levels drop, 90 percent of women will experience up to eight years of irregular menstrual periods, hot flashes, and mood swings before menopause (peri-menopause), which occurs, on average, at age 51. For men there is a decreased production of testosterone, and for both sexes, here are the symptoms:

increased body fat

decreased strength/mass of muscles

fragile bones

decreased body hair where you want it, and increase in hair on the face ears and nose.

swelling/tenderness in the breast tissue

hot flashes in women, and decreased temperature regulation in men

increased fatigue

effects on cholesterol metabolism

"The really frightening thing about middle age is the knowledge that you'll grow out of it" – Doris Day

In Your 50s

In your 50s, the first serious signs of aging occur: memory loss may be more pronounced, and changes in the skin and your physique become noticeable. Starting at 50, many people begin to lose height; it can be very slight, and gradual, but just be aware that this can happen. I am a half-inch shorter than I was just 5 years ago. Abdominal weight gain, sagging and dry skin, the hair on your head thins, then appears on your face and in your nose and ears. More than a quarter of people between 50 and 64 are obese; nearly 44 percent are overweight. Men and women both feel they are

Marvelous Menopause

This is the time in a woman's life when the ability to bear children ends and the next phase of life begins. For me, the loss of fertility was sad, but it also brought on the ability to be fully free with who and what I am both personally and professionally. This should be embraced and celebrated by all.

Yet instead, as a society, both men and women are scared and uninformed about the totally natural process of menopause. Even though this transition is natural, and women are often happier at this stage in their lives than ever, the mere mention of menopause implies loss of femininity, beauty, and sexual desire.

I like to focus on the positives. The concern of becoming pregnant is gone, so there is a newfound freedom sexually, and that sense of fierce competition in life starts to dwindle, making friendships easier and more meaningful.

During peri-menopause and early menopause, women may suffer from hot flashes, sweating, sleep disturbances and memory loss. Although temporary in most cases, this can be exhausting, resulting in a negative impact on our quality of life at home and work. Due to menopause being viewed as negative, and reducing one's value to society, women will tend to isolate and minimize what is happening, which leads to anxiety, depression, and poor self-esteem.

This is the time for reaching out and embracing help. I find when I seek out other women I can share my menopause concerns with I feel less alone, and my confidence soars! We all feel the fear of being left behind, passed over for promotions and other opportunities at work, but the more we talk about it with others it will normalize and hopefully dispel the myths surrounding aging women. →

Many men, (sorry guys!) buy into the stereotype of a menopausal woman being emotionally frazzled and intellectually compromised so they tend to discriminate against older females. This is especially prevalent in the workplace. I have experienced this firsthand, and it left me feeling lost, baffled, and defeated.

The catch-22 here is that negative thinking, anxiety and stress, can make the symptoms worse. When menopause is embraced as natural phase of the life cycle and women are empowered, everyone will benefit. Through thoughtful changes in exercise, food selections, and self-care including meditation and rest, the temporary side effects of this natural process can be managed with grace and calm.

While some medications may help with the symptoms of early menopause, some such as hormone replacement therapy (HRT) have been stopped or limited due to scientific studies that show any benefits are far outweighed by increased risk of blood clot, stroke, breast, or uterine cancer.

Instead, try this Eat Well Tip: add a lot of soy products to your diet at this time! Soy isoflavones have been shown to mimic estrogen, so try drinking soymilk, eating black or green soybeans, enjoying soy meats and soy cheese, using different kinds of tofu in recipes that call for eggs or dairy ingredients. If you really don't like any soy foods, look for menopause supplements in your natural foods store, as many contain soy isoflavones. Many women have found that using soy in this way helps to reduce the symptoms such as hot flashes and night sweats, making the transition that much easier. Once you're over the transition period, you can use soy products as you desire.

starting to look old, and both sexes are very susceptible to buying "anti-aging" products, with promises getting slicker all the time!

More than half of people over 50 report some memory loss such as forgetting names and misplacing keys. I get very upset when this happens, and I keep looking for ways to be organized as I go about my day. The other main complaint is a dramatic decline in vision. These usually don't result from illness but from normal, age-related changes in the brain and body. Simple steps like taking time to remember things and making lists can help, and always wear your glasses or contacts! If you stay on top of it you are less likely to have an injury, or hurt someone else. I go every year for an eye exam, and upgrade my prescriptions as needed.

Starting at age 50, your risk for all chronic diseases goes up, especially heart disease. The risk of common cancers increase. Schedule screening tests for breast cancer, cervical cancer, prostate cancer, and colon cancer, the second-leading cause of cancer deaths. If you have a strong family history of a particular disease, go get screened at 40. These tests are very routine and easy to schedule, and early detection leads to the best outcomes for any needed treatments.

Eat well tip
As we age, it seems the struggle to eat right and take care of ourselves is contrary to the idea of just doing what we want, when we want, and enjoying ourselves. A glass of wine, a rich meal, and a creamy dessert are all wonderful to experience! All those years we spent dieting and worrying about what people think of us are over, yet we still need to pay attention to our wellness into old age. I suggest taking one day a week for yourself to relax, eat something indulgent, and savor the moment. (Not every day! Just one day...)

Other health concerns in the 40s and 50s include stiffness in the body's muscles, tendons, ligaments and joints. We start to feel banged up very easily, and take longer to recover from strains and sprains, especially if you are a "weekend warrior" (someone who engages in vigorous physical activity on Saturday and Sunday after being inactive most of the week). Instead of slowing down, try to adjust and keep active — maybe allowing yourself to enjoy a slightly lower level of performance. The risks associated with a sedentary lifestyle far exceeds the risks of physical activity. Regular exercise, including weight training and stretching, keeps tissues supple, stabilizes joints, and helps prevent excess weight gain.

In Your 60s

By the time we reach 60, hopefully your work life will begin to wind down, because our hearts, ears, and eyes start to deteriorate, and arthritis starts to set in. Bad health habits become a real concern as now is when the irreversible damage occurs. The cardiovascular system becomes less efficient during exercise because the heart's function and oxygen exchange declines, and we often sleep less than when we were younger, giving the body less time to recuperate and regenerate overnight. For all of these reasons, it is critical to engage in very healthy habits as you enter your 60s. Women have a distinct advantage over men in that they live longer, especially if they exercise. Highly active 65-year-old women are expected to live nearly six years longer than their sedentary counterparts.

Hearing. About one-third of Americans older than 65 have trouble hearing. Vertigo may also set in, which can be caused by inner ear problems. Have your ears checked as part of your annual routine.

Brain. According to the Alzheimer's Association, one in 10 people over 65 has Alzheimer's disease. Alzheimer's disease (AD), is a chronic neurodegenerative disease that usually starts slowly and gradually worsens over the course of time. There can be worsening of symptoms anywhere from a few months to a few years. (More info on Alzheimer's and dementia in the next chapter.)

Pill Concerns. Americans over 65 take an average of four prescription drugs a day, plus an unknown number of over-the-counter medications such as pain relievers, anti-inflammatories,

A Note about Arthritis:

After a few years of dealing with decreasing mobility in my left hip and difficulty running, I convinced my doctor to do a scan and was diagnosed with severe degenerative joint disease. His first response was, "if you keep this pace up, you are headed for a hip replacement!" I was devastated, thinking there was nothing I could do. After re-grouping and doing a lot of research, I learned that Arthritis is a very common condition, and it seems to have a strong hereditary component. Arthritis in itself is not the disease; it is a catch-all term that defines joint pain, degenerative joint disease, and the inflammation that results from a multitude of disorders. In my case it presents as stiffness and loss of flexibility.

According to the Arthritis Association (www.arthritis.org), there are more than 100 different types of arthritis and related conditions. More than 50 million adults have arthritis, and it is the leading cause of disability in America. It is more common among women and the elderly. So many of my peers are suffering with some form of arthritis, yet there are now so many advances in treatment.

If you are experiencing swelling, pain, stiffness and decreased range of motion in the areas around your joints, I urge you to get evaluated by an orthopedic surgeon. Keep in mind that the symptoms may come and go, and vary from mild, to moderate or severe. They may stay the same for years, or get worse over time. Severe arthritis can result in chronic pain, inability to do daily activities and make it difficult to walk or climb stairs. Arthritis can cause permanent joint changes and is often only detected by a scan or X-ray. Like anything else, the earlier you address it the better. I am choosing to treat mine with →

physical therapy, walking, and heavy weight training to keep my muscles strong. While I may not run marathons as fast as I once did, I am sure to remain active and flexible.

Ironically, while arthritis can make it hard to painful to move, the most common prescription for it is: exercise! By staying (or becoming) active, our body's natural synovial fluid increases in the joints, helping to lubricate them and move more smoothly and easily with less pain. Don't let fear stop you from being physically active, check with a health professional such as a physical therapist or personal trainer who specializes in older adults or arthritis treatment about the best exercises for you.

And don't think that non-impact activities such as swimming or elliptical are necessarily better for you! The impact from running and jumping actually helps you to maintain stronger bones, and combat another bane of growing older, which is osteoporosis and fractures. Again, check with your health professional about what is best for you.

antacids, antihistamines, diarrhea or constipation remedies, allergy pills, cough suppressants, eyedrops, and more — as well as multiple herbal or vitamin supplements. But taken in the wrong combination, a cocktail of drugs can harm instead of heal. Older people are particularly vulnerable to unanticipated drug interactions because of changes in their bodies, including muscle loss, fat gain and diminished liver and kidney function. The changes might require a dosage adjustment and greater vigilance. Consult your doctor or pharmacist before adding or changing your vitamin and medication routine. I subscribe to the old adage, only take medication that is absolutely necessary.

In Your 70s

Entering into your 70s! As physical and cognitive abilities continue their slow decline, there is an increasing need to exercise the body

visit, and enjoy connections in the community such as weekly religious services, social service activities, and like-minded social media groups.

Stay physically active: "Use it or lose it" rings true here. Do something every day — from walking around the neighborhood to senior exercise class, especially something aerobic — to maintain cardiovascular health. As noted above, weight training and impact activities become more important, as putting stress onto muscles transfers to bones and improves bone health. Balance ("proprioception") and flexibility are also critical in advanced years: often, once someone in their 70s or 80s takes a fall, and breaks a hip, recovery is very difficult, and many never fully recuperate. This is when it is important to check the house for things that might cause a trip and fall, such as small throw rugs, extension cords, or slippery floors.

"Walking is the best possible exercise. Habituate yourself to walk very far" – Thomas Jefferson

A study of nursing-home residents in their 80s and 90s showed it's never too late to reap the benefits of exercise. After 10 weeks, octogenarians on a weight-training program boosted their walking speed and increased their strength by 113 percent. Some even tossed aside their walkers for the first time in years. If you are unable to stand or walk, whether it is temporary or permanent, see the list of choices provided for seated exercises in Chapter 6, where I discuss fitness for life. As we move along the road — "Truckin'" as the Grateful Dead song title says — learning and changing and growing, I often think about their greatest hits album, which they entitled "What a long strange trip it's been." Indeed it has!

Interactive Chapter Review

How and Why We Age: As we age, genetic inheritance becomes less of a factor and environment and lifestyle become more important.

Do you think that being old means you will be sick and frail? Is it inevitable that there is a dramatic decline in physical *and mental abilities? Do you think longevity is solely the result of a genetic lottery, or can you do things to enhance and extend your life?*

Do you worry about memory loss? Have you started to experience this? How do you deal with it? Can you be more organized? Would making lists help you? In what areas?

How is your vision? Do you wear glasses? Contacts? Have you had lasik surgery? Remember, don't squint, it's bad for your eyes and causes wrinkles!

Speaking of wrinkles... have you tried all the "anti-aging" lotions and potions? Cosmetic surgery? Do you avoid the sun, or are you a sun-worshipper despite the proven dangers of UV rays, both in terms of skin cancer and its aging effects? Do you have a regular, simple skin care regimen that you follow consistently? Remember: the best thing you can do for your skin is be happy!

Aging Through the Decades. *What do you remember of your 20s? Party time? Or stress from worrying about jobs, relationships, money, the future? Did you make poor decisions regarding drinking and drug use, promiscuity, irresponsible behaviors? Do you miss those days, or are you just as glad they're behind you? Did you feel invincible, and that you didn't have to worry about the effects of aging? Did you eat well and stay active, or did you ignore those concerns and start putting on weight?*

Did you start to see signs of aging in your 30s? What were they — grey hair, fine lines, reduced muscle and increased fat storage? Slowing metabolism? Did diabetes affect you?

What about in your 40s? Did advancing signs of age start to appear? Age-related diseases such as cancer and heart disease? Vision and hearing loss? Did you continue or take up physical activity? Achieve some career stability? How did you manage stress from juggling child-rearing and caring for aging parents simultaneously? Did your sexual drive change — in either direction? What about the other changes associated with a drop in testosterone levels and/or the onset of menopause? Did you do anything to address these?

What signs of aging in your 50s have you experienced, or do you worry about? Memory loss, changes in skin and hair, loss of height, hearing and vision issues, abdominal weight gain, increase of chronic diseases, pain and stiffness? Do you think you are susceptible to buying "anti-aging" products if the claims are seductive enough? Will you or have you scheduled the screening tests for serious diseases? Have you started or do you continue to lead an active lifestyle? Do you take one day (just one!) each week just to enjoy and indulge?

Have poor health choices earlier in life started to manifest in your 60s? Can you make changes to address those, such as quitting smoking, reducing alcohol consumption, increasing your activity level, and making better food choices? Do you worry about brain, eyes, hearing functions? Are you taking multiple prescription medications?

Counteract the continued physical and mental decline of the 70s with increased physical and mental exercise! Start to prepare for elder care and after-life planning. Ensure you continue to enjoy nutritious and energizing food by caring for your dental health, while reducing consumption due to reduced exercise and slowing metabolism.

Do you think you will make it into your 80s? Why/why not? The older you are, the more your life expectancy increases. Continue to celebrate your birthdays and do what it takes to stay strong and sharp. Maintain your appearance, continue your connections with friends and family, engage with social groups in your community and online.

What will you do to remain physically active? Have you taken steps to reduce causes for trips and falls in your home? Are you unable to stand or workout for long periods of time? Consider a seated workout or chair yoga. (See Chapter 6 for details)

Chapter 4
Medical Tests and Physical Assessments

Regardless of your chronological age, and how you have lived up until now, you need to take full responsibility for your own healthcare and well-being going forward. There is so much information available to us now: reputable (and not-so-reputable) health websites on the internet, drug commercials on TV, your best friend had such-and-such treatment, your second cousin had an obscure disease and his doctor told him blah-blah-blah. You can research and self-diagnose all you want, but you won't know your own health status without going to a doctor and getting your own health checked out now.

To prepare for your appointment, write down your symptoms and concerns ahead of time, and discuss with your doctor any changes in your body that you might be experiencing. No matter how minor it may seem to you, it could help the doctor in evaluating you. Lastly, don't lie to the doctor or withhold information, because you will only hurt yourself in the long run. It is probable that your doctor has heard and seen things far worse than what you are presenting.

Please know that you have every right to interview several doctors before you choose who you will be working with. I have experienced prejudice and pre-conceived notions that doctors had towards me, which led to my having to change health care providers midway through treatment. When I was diagnosed with arthritis in my hip. It took almost a year to get a doctor to order the necessary tests for me because I always present as very healthy and fit, they just assumed it was tight muscles. As the Robert Palmer song title says, *"Doctor, Doctor, give me the news."*

"You are in a partnership with your doctor, and it needs to be a give and take"

Obesity, arthritis, alcoholism, and heart disease are just some of the conditions that are still regarded by some health care providers as a result of character flaws, laziness, and personal neglect. One friend of mine, who has a high BMI despite being extremely active, is always told by doctors first thing that she has to lose weight. She has learned to ask what advice they would give a thinner person who has the same condition? Surely they wouldn't tell them to lose weight. That way she obtains more in-depth advice and information than simply to go on a diet.

Once you have chosen who you will be working with, it can be beneficial to take a family member or friend along on your doctor's appointment to take notes. You may not hear everything that the doctor is telling you because of anxiety or feeling overwhelmed — and most of us hear only what we want to hear, so we miss a lot. Plus, having the support of another person to talk to, travel with, or get appointments and medications confirmed for you is invaluable. Most friends or family members would be pleased to support you in this way, to make sure you listen closely — and fully absorb — the best medical advice available.

"If I'd known I was going to live this long, I'd have taken better care of myself" - Anonymous

Medical Specialists

Here are the doctors and tests you need for evaluation. You can take this book with you to ensure the doctor is being thorough, and to remind yourself of what you need to look for.

Internist/General Practitioner. Get a basic evaluation first. This includes your weight, height, blood pressure, and resting heart rate. The next level of testing should include glucose tolerance testing for diabetes, electrocardiogram for the heart function, and complete blood tests for an overall evaluation of your health status. Your GP (general practitioner) may refer you to other specialists including a cardiologist, pulmonologist, rheumatologist, endocrinologist, allergist, oncologist, neurologist, dermatologist, orthopedist, etc., depending on symptoms or test results.

Ear, Nose and Throat (ENT). Get a hearing test! A majority of Baby Boomers and beyond suffer from hearing loss, due to all those loud concerts of our youth. One of the most overlooked health issues is hearing loss. This can affect balance, which may lead to falls and serious injury. And missing out on conversation and interaction may cause you to feel isolated and depressed without even realizing it. Left uncorrected, it can even hasten the onset of dementia. Most hearing loss can be managed with hearing aids. The biggest hurdle is usually getting people to admit their hearing loss and get treatment. My family has a pre-disposition towards hearing loss, and we all have spent countless hours screaming at each other to be heard.

Continual or regular sore throat, coughing, throat clearing, or nose-blowing may also be signs of other conditions worth addressing proactively.

Ophthalmologist. General vision, glaucoma test, and prescription update for glasses or contacts. It's probably time to talk to the eye doctor about getting nonprescription magnifying glasses for reading, too. You may develop floaters, which are black squiggly lines in your vision from the gel in your eyes hardening, which is common in middle age. It is not dangerous unless you are seeing flashing lights and/or your vision is disrupted, which may be symptoms of a detached retina. Starting in your 40s you need to be tested for macular degeneration and cataracts. Vision decline can put you at risk for falls. It also can limit reading and travel, which can lead to isolation and depression.

"Only floss the teeth you want to keep"

Dentist. Get X-rays to see if you have any new cavities. Have your teeth cleaned every 4-6 months for gum health, and have your bite checked. Your teeth shift as you age and can cause chewing and digestive problems. You may be seeing a lot of adults now with braces because they are trying to correct this and avoid getting dentures late in life. If you teeth are yellowing, think about veneers or cosmetic whitening, which is relatively inexpensive and will give your confidence a boost. I got Invisalign a few years ago to correct my bite which was changing due to age related shifting of my teeth. Not only did it correct it, my teeth look great!

To manage your dental health at home, brush and floss your teeth every day. According to Michael Rozien, MD, author of *The Real Age Diet*, you can add 6-7 years to your life just by flossing your teeth regularly. My favorite dental hygienist once said something to me I remember every day: "Only floss the teeth you want to keep!"

Dental work can be very expensive. One solution is to go to a nearby dental school and see if they have a teaching clinic. You may have students work on you, they are well supervised by well-respected senior dentists, and the care is great! If you are missing teeth, look into bridges, dentures, and implants, not only for cosmetic reasons but to help with chewing. Digestion begins in the mouth, and to maintain good nutrition as we age, we want to be able to chew and enjoy a variety of hard and crunchy foods, and fully absorb the nutrients of everything we eat.

Dermatologist. Ask the doctor about the latest in skincare and skin cancer prevention. Be sure to use 30 SPF sunscreen on any exposed skin whenever you go outside, especially for prolonged periods of time — and remember the tops of your ears. Avoid tanning, whether outdoors or on a tanning bed, as this has been proven to cause premature skin aging and skin cancer.

Get any moles and spots checked at least once a year, and learn the "ABCDE" of skin cancer prevention: Asymmetry, Border, Color, Diameter, and Evolving (changing). Benign moles are usually symmetrical, with a clear border, single color, small diameter, and do not change over time, while melanomas are often asymmetrical, with no defined border, multiple colors, cover a wider area and tend to grow and change over time.

I found a tiny black dot on my knee that turned out to be the beginning stages of Melanoma. Early detection made it possible for me to catch it in time, and be cancer free. While skin cancer is the main concern for all of us as we age, you may have other skin conditions that you've been hesitant to share with your doctor, including dry skin, itching, chafing, adult acne, psoriasis or eczema. There are treatments and medications that can reduce the annoyance or discomfort associated with these issues, you just have to ask for help.

"If someone wishes for good health, one must first ask oneself if he is ready to do away with the reasons for his illness. Only then is it possible to help him." — Hippocrates

Gynecologist/Urologist. Cancer screening and tests for all sexually transmitted diseases are necessary at any age if you (and/or your partner) are sexually active. Over 40, for women mammograms are recommended for breast health, and for men prostate cancer screening is mandatory starting at 50. This includes having a blood test called the PSA (prostate specific antigen) level checked because when this is elevated it could indicate disease. The other essential exam is a physical exam of the rectum to look for any abnormalities in the prostate gland. Hormone levels for both sexes is worth checking as well.

As with the dermatologist, don't be embarrassed to ask about issues you may have with itching, discharge, odor, dryness, discomfort or pain during intercourse — your gynecologist is familiar with all of these issues and may have suggestions to help you with them.

Gastroenterologist. As you age, your chances of colon cancer increase. At 50, it is highly recommended to have a colonoscopy. You should have it done younger if you have a family history of the disease. There is a new test out now called Cologuard which is a way of giving a stool sample at home and mailing it into a lab. Start there to have a baseline and some peace of mind!

Again, document and discuss any symptoms that may trouble you, including abdominal pain or excess gas when you eat certain foods. If you have recurrent or serious reflux (heartburn), diarrhea, constipation, nausea, indigestion — don't just treat these with over-the-counter medications, talk to your doctor to discuss possible ways to prevent these issues.

Chiropractor. Get a spinal adjustment, not just to treat back pain or injury, but to function at your best every day. Chiropractic is minimally invasive, and really helps you to feel great. Dr. Elizabeth Greenberg, DC, a chiropractor and Wellness advisor in New York City states, "If you think about the fact that everything in your body is controlled by your brain, from your conscious muscle movements to unconscious body processes such as digestion — and realizing that the brain's signals are all transmitted through the spinal cord — ensuring that your spine is properly aligned is important for your full body functioning at its best."

Therapeutic Massage is also a great way to help you reduce muscle tension and be more relaxed and positive throughout your day.

Orthopedist/Podiatrist. Any walking or gait issues can cause kinetic chain problems, so it's a good idea to address issues from flat feet to high arches, and prevent knee pain, lower back pain, and other common problems from arising as we grow older. Arthritis, rheumatism and other joint pains are often alleviated by increasing regular activity such as walking, swimming, and biking. Get any and all severe joint pain checked out before taking up physical activity to ensure your safety. Exercise is so important to keep us healthy and happy, it is important to care for our orthopedic health so can continue — or start — to be fit and active for our overall well-being.

Physical Therapy is a much gentler, more natural approach to address underlying causes of pain or discomfort rather than treating symptoms through medication or surgery. In fact, the recovery time for treatment of many orthopedic conditions is the same with or without surgery, and both require physical therapy to achieve full range of motion. Sometimes it is best to treat injury with therapy alone.

Preventing Falls

Falls are more common as we age, and become very serious after age 65. Many older people never fully recover from injuries that occur as a result of falls. Take these steps to prevent falls:

> Correct poor vision by wearing prescribed glasses or contacts

> Check your hearing to be sure there are no inner ear issues that might cause balance problems

> Wear shoes with adequate heel support and non-slip soles, and avoid extremely high heels

Exercise to increase strength, coordination and balance (proprioception); specifically practice balancing in order to maintain and improve this critical skill

Talk to your doctor about decreasing medications that impair balance

Use canes or walkers if needed

Take extra care, watch your step, and use handrails on stairs and ramps, especially if they are uneven

Consider hip-protection pads if you are at risk for falling

Avoid drug use or excessive alcohol consumption

Eliminate hazards such as loose electrical cords and throw rugs in your home

Make sure rooms and hallways are well lit with nightlights that are placed along the walls

Dementia and Alzheimer's

While these may be two of the most dreaded words in the English language for those of us growing older, they should be addressed with knowledge rather than fear. This may be particularly difficult for those of us who have lost loved ones due to these conditions, or are currently caring for aging parents or grandparents who suffer from the worst symptoms, including lack of recognition of loved ones, uncontrolled emotions and bodily functions, getting lost or confused, and more. Dementia is a blanket term for illnesses that cause memory loss, confusion, personality changes and a decline in one's ability to function and do basic tasks that were once easy.

There are two general types of dementias, and 5 types of dementia that are of unknown origin or a result on another disease that affects the brain:

Alzheimer's, which is when proteins in the brain get tangled around brain cells causing difficulty in brain cells to communicate with each other properly. There is a hereditary component, but there is

Alzheimer's is the cause of most dementia cases, but not all dementia results in Alzheimer's. The most common early symptom is difficulty in remembering recent events, short term memory becomes severely diminished. When someone is constantly repeating themselves or asking the same questions over and over, it might be time for an evaluation. One reason that it is so difficult to diagnose early on is because the person will often remember all of the details of an event from 50 years ago, so it seems that the memory is intact.

As the disease advances, symptoms can include problems with language, disorientation and getting lost on a familiar route, both walking and driving. As a person's condition declines, they will have mood swings, loss of motivation and personal hygiene often suffers, Another symptom is withdrawal from family and society, and behavioral problems ensue, much like a defiant child. Gradually, bodily functions are lost, ultimately leading to death. Although the speed of progression can vary, the typical life expectancy following diagnosis is three to nine years.

no guarantee that you will or will not get Alzheimer's. A healthy lifestyle will absolutely reduce your risk of being afflicted with this.

Vascular dementia is a type of dementia that appears to have many of the same symptoms as Alzheimer's. It is more treatable because it is a direct result of insufficient blood flow to the brain. Blood flow is affected by clogged arteries and the interruption of this blood flow can cause areas of dead tissues, resulting in mini strokes which is a direct cause of dementia. Keeping your heart and lungs fit is a big part of reducing the likelihood of vascular dementia.

Mixed Dementia is dementia that is caused by more than one type of dementia at the same time.

Lewy Body is the third most common form of dementia. It is caused by abnormally folded proteins in the brain.

Parkinson's and Huntington's diseases can also have co-existing dementia as the disease progresses.

This gets back to same general guidelines to improve all conditions as we age: eating well, exercising, getting frequent checkups, and engaging your mind with challenging and rewarding activities all help us to age well.

The Importance of Sleep

It is really important to develop a consistent sleep schedule. With age this seems to be harder and harder to come by. There are many factors that prevent us from having a good night's sleep, but by making sleep and resting a priority you will fare batter later in life.

Insufficient sleep is detrimental to your overall heath and can contribute to an early death. According to an article by Camille Peri at WebMD, lack of sleep, and poor quality sleep can lead to accidents and injuries at the workplace, compromised judgment, and impairs attention, alertness, concentration, reasoning, and problem solving.

"Every night, before you go to bed, know you will wake up to a new day with new possibilities"

We always hear that adults, both male and female, require 7 to 8 hours of sleep per night. Some people can get away 5-6 hours, or in the case of teens, they may require as much as 9-10 hours of sleep each day in order to feel fully rested and mentally sharp. I know from personal experience lack of sleep negatively effects my concentration, moods and ability to make sound decisions. It can be just as detrimental as being drunk or high while trying to function throughout the day.

Here is a breakdown of the sleep cycles you need to feel fully rested when you wake up. Also note that sleep works to restore your body and consolidate your thoughts and memories. A good night's sleep will help you store and remember what you learned and experienced each day, and will contribute to the efficiency of your long term memory.

Stage 1. This is the lightest stage of sleep, the transition phase, where you feel yourself falling asleep without effort. If you were to forget about the alarm clock and allow yourself to wake up naturally, Stage 1 sleep would be the last stage before you fully wake up. You don't spend too much time in Stage 1 sleep, typically five to 10 minutes, just enough to allow your body to slow down and your muscles to relax.

Stage 2. This is still considered light sleep, yet brain activity starts to slow down, as well as your heart rate and breathing. Your body temperature lowers and you start to reach a state of total relaxation in preparation for the deeper sleep to come.

Stage 3. This is the start of deep sleep, also known as slow wave sleep. During this stage, your brain waves are slow "delta waves," although there may still be short bursts of faster of brain activity known as "beta-waves." If you were to get awakened suddenly during this stage, you would be groggy and confused, and find it difficult to focus at first.

Stage 4. Of the five stages of sleep, this is the one when you experience your deepest sleep of the night. Your brain only shows delta-wave (slow wave) activity, and it's difficult to wake someone up when they're in Stage 4 of sleep.

Stages 3 and 4 can last anywhere from 5 to 15 minutes each, but the first deep sleep of the night is more likely to be an hour or so. This is the time when the body does most of its repair work and regeneration.

Stage 5. This is the stage of sleep when you dream. It is also called "active sleep" or REM sleep, which stands for Rapid Eye Movements (REM).

During REM sleep, the muscles in your arms and legs will go through periods of paralysis. Scientists speculate that this may be nature's way of protecting us from acting out our dreams. The first period of REM sleep of the night usually begins about 90 minutes after you start drifting off, and lasts for about 10 minutes. As the night passes, the periods of REM sleep become longer, with the final episode lasting an hour or so. For a healthy adult, Stage 5 occurs for about 20 to 25% of the time you are sleeping, and decreases with age.

Scientists and researchers are continually learning more about the mechanics and physiological effects of sleep, and what happens during the five stages of sleep. Sleep deprivation can result in lower libido and less interest in sex. Depleted energy, sleepiness, and increased tension may be largely to blame. Sleep apnea, a respiratory problem that interrupts sleep, may be another factor in the sexual slump, according to a 2002 study published in the *Journal of Clinical Endocrinology & Metabolism*. Since sleep apnea interrupts the flow of oxygen to the rest of the body, it can have serious adverse effects on heart health, brain health, and even cause daytime drowsiness.

"Though sleep is called our best friend, it is a friend who often keeps us waiting!" – Jules Verne

According to some estimates, 90% of people with insomnia — a sleep disorder characterized by trouble falling and staying asleep — also have other health conditions. Over time, lack of sleep and sleep disorders can contribute to anxiety and depression.

Most people have experienced sallow skin and puffy eyes after a few nights of missed sleep. Indeed, chronic sleep loss can lead to lackluster skin, fine lines, and dark circles under the eyes.

Trying to keep your memory sharp? Get plenty of sleep. In 2009, American and French researchers determined that brain events called "sharp wave ripples" are responsible for consolidating memory. These ripples also transfer learned information from the hippocampus to the neocortex of the brain, where long-term memories are stored. Sharp wave ripples occur mostly during the deepest levels of sleep.

**"Sleep that knits up the ravelled sleeve of care
The death of each day's life, sore labour's bath
Balm of hurt minds, great nature's second course,
Chief nourisher in life's feast."
— William Shakespeare, Macbeth**

In the "Whitehall II Study," British researchers looked at how sleep patterns affected the mortality of more than 10,000 British civil servants over two decades. The results, published in 2007, showed that those who had cut their sleep from seven to five hours or fewer a night nearly doubled their risk of death from all causes. In particular, lack of sleep doubled the risk of death from cardiovascular disease.

Lack of sleep can affect our interpretation of events. This hurts our ability to make sound judgments because we may not assess situations accurately and act on them wisely. Sleep-deprived people seem to be especially prone to poor judgment when it comes to assessing what lack of sleep is doing to them.

Not getting enough sleep can be downright dangerous. The National Sleep Foundation's 2008 *Sleep in America* poll showed that 36% of Americans drive drowsy or fall asleep while driving. In our increasingly fast-paced world, functioning on less sleep has become a kind of badge of honor. But sleep specialists say if you think you're doing fine on less sleep, you're probably wrong. And if you work in a profession where it's important to be able to judge your level of functioning, this can be a big problem.

According to Philip Gehrman, PhD, CBSM at University of Pennsylvania, "Studies show that over time, people who are getting six hours of sleep, instead of seven or eight, begin to feel that they've adapted to that sleep deprivation — they've gotten used to it, but if you look at how they actually do on tests of mental alertness and performance, they continue to go downhill. So there's a point in sleep deprivation when we lose touch with how impaired we are."

You don't want to sleep too much, either. Seven to eight hours is the "sweet spot" as shown in a 22-year-long study of twins, with those who sleep less than 7 hours or more than 8 hours per night having an increased rate of death by 17-24 percent. Using sleep medications also increases mortality risk by about one-third.

Helpful Hints on Getting a Good Night's Sleep

We all don't fall asleep immediately when we hit the pillow, so you may want to increase the time you spend unwinding. Get in bed, shut off the electronics and read or do a puzzle. It really helps with relaxing the body so that you will sleep more soundly.

The National Sleep Foundation notes: "In general, exercising regularly makes it easier to fall asleep and contributes to sounder sleep. However, exercising sporadically or right before going to bed will make falling asleep more difficult." It is very important to include rest and recovery time in any exercise program.

If you need to wake up really early — let's say, so you can get your exercise in before work — and want to have at least 7 hours of sleep, add an extra half hour to your bedtime. For example, if you want to get up at 6:00 a.m. try to be in bed by 10-10:30 p.m. Pay attention to how long it takes you to fall asleep, and time it accordingly.

> **"A good laugh and a long sleep are the best cures in the doctor's book." - Irish Proverb**

Many people have success using various bedtime routines, including soft music or white noise machines that can help lull you to sleep. If you have difficulty with insomnia, consult your doctor, pharmacist, or natural food store for natural remedies, such as valerian root, chamomile, St. John's Wort, or melatonin, or using aromatherapy with lavender oil, Melissa, or lemon balm. It's best to avoid over the counter or prescription sleep medication if possible, as this can upset your natural circadian rhythms, and may cause drug dependency.

Stop Smoking Cigarettes!

Smoking cigarettes was widely accepted in society all over the world for many years. I can tell you from personal experience for many people in my age group, kids growing up in the '60s and '70s, smoking cigarettes enhanced the feeling of fitting in and being cool. The song title *"Smokin' in the Boys Room"* by Brownsville Station was descriptive of our teenage years. The teachers told us to stop, we heard the warnings, yet no one knew how really harmful smoking is for us and those around us. I stopped smoking at 21, and sadly many of my friends who continued all had health problems later on.

So if you smoke, stop now. Not only does it compromise your health, secondhand smoke hurts everyone around you. Smoking increases your risk of Alzheimer's by 50%. But our powers of recovery are amazing: if a smoker quits by age 50, by the time he or she reaches 64, his or her risk of dying is similar to that of someone who never smoked. I often hear from older people, "I made it this long, why quit now?" The answer is, because its harmful for you and everyone around you — and yes, quitting now, even after many years of smoking, will still have positive health effects.

In general, the desire for a cigarette is actually the desire for more air — try taking long, slow, deep breaths to quiet the urge to pick up a cigarette. This also has a calming, meditative effect that one is usually seeking from the nicotine in cigarettes — but you can actually get from deep breathing, not from chemicals. If you want something to put in your mouth, try strong-flavored toothpicks, like licorice, cinnamon, or peppermint.

One friend of mine had success in quitting smoking by putting a drop of strong mouthwash into an empty water-based cigarette filter, available at drug stores. When she wanted a cigarette, she took a drag on the filter, and the little "hit" of mouthwash gave her that numb feeling on the tip of her tongue like a cigarette. There are also mild anti-depressive drugs that are prescribed to help with nicotine withdrawal, as well as nicotine replacements such as gum and patches — but be careful about becoming as reliant on these items as were on the cigarettes themselves. These are tools to wean you off of smoking, not alternatives like the new "e-cigarettes" which are being shown to have their own health concerns.

Let them go. It feels wonderful not to have to smoke!

Decrease Alcohol Consumption

The current science shows that red wine can be good for us. This is because there are helpful antioxidants in the skin of red grapes that helps reduce the risk of heart disease. Keep in mind that it is the grapes, not the alcohol, that has the health benefits! You get the same benefit from red or purple grape juice, which is family friendly and can be consumed even by those who do not drink for other reasons. This is why white wine — or white grape juice — is not touted as a "health food."

If you drink alcohol excessively, more than one glass every day, then evaluate its usefulness in your life. Despite the confidence and relaxant effect it gives you, are you aware that alcohol or other substances cloud your judgment on just about everything? Will you enjoy the evening just as much if you have, say, just one drink instead of three or four? Studies have shown that women should limit drinks to one a day, and men to two a day — and there is nothing wrong with cutting out alcohol use altogether. For men, alcohol can impair the quality and quantity of sperm, reduce testosterone and contribute to erectile dysfunction. And no one, of course, should ever drink and drive.

If you think it's difficult to reduce your alcohol consumption, either physically or socially, you may consider seeking outside support. Sometimes it seems like we'd stand out like a sore thumb if we attend a social event without an alcoholic drink in hand. However, most people don't actually notice what you're drinking; you can always have a sparkling water or juice, and no one will be the wiser. Remember, many people do not drink alcohol for a variety of reasons, including religious dictates, dietary guidelines, medication conflicts, sports training, pregnancy, or recovery. You do not need to explain or justify why you are choosing not to drink, just say, "No, thank you," "Not tonight," or "Not for me, thanks."

Another thing to be aware of is that alcoholic tendencies may arise at any age. Many seniors have alcoholism set in once they have retired or become empty nesters. Being alone and losing one's daily goals can lead to loneliness and isolation. Depression may set in, and that's when excessive drinking can start. There is an acronym that many recovery groups use when the going gets tough: HALT!

Eat well tip

The trend towards drinking alcoholic beverages when socializing has skyrocketed. With an ever increasing menu of specialty cocktails, and the explosion of niche breweries and exotic wineries throughout the world, consuming alcohol is at an all-time high! Enjoy it, experience the flavors, but drink responsibly. 1 to 2 drinks maximum!! If you feel you are overdoing it and cannot stop, reach out for help.

At the same time, many trendy eateries are offering specialty "mocktails" with flavors, seasonings, shrubs and bitters — but no alcohol. Try one of these, or just some soda water with fruit, to keep your friends company without overdoing the alcohol.

There's no need to be self-conscious if you don't indulge: people have dozens of reasons for avoiding alcohol, it might interfere with medications they are taking, they have to drive later, they are preparing for an athletic event or academic exam or work presentation, it could be against religious beliefs, or they're just not in the mood. You never have to explain why you say, "No, thanks, not for me."

Don't allow yourself to get too Hungry, Angry, Lonely or Tired. This is another reason why social interaction and taking care of yourself is so important.

Odds and Ends

As we age, there is a tendency to think that every ache and pain might be a life threatening emergency. By and large, however, we are a lot healthier than we think — and those little aches and pains are just aches and pains, not symptoms of a serious health crisis.

Our bodies have certain unexplained symptoms that frighten us but are really just natural mechanisms that help regulate our equilibrium and keep us in touch with how we function. Unfortunately, they tend to occur when we least expect it, and when we are in a situation that can cause embarrassment.

Here are some simple explanations for those strange and funny symptoms that we all have:

Excessive itching. Itching is usually due to an allergic reaction to scented soaps, fabrics, plants, and animals. Extreme dryness in arid hot weather (or with excessive radiator heat in the wintertime), and excessive exercising can also cause itching. One way to keep this to a minimum is to use moisturizing shampoos and body creams after showering. If it persists, get it checked out.

Excessive sweating (hyperhidrosis). This can occur on any part of your body, not just your underarms, including hands and feet. Often this can be reduced with the use of antiperspirants or powders. Some people with truly excessive sweating — especially athletes, for whom it may affect performance — treat this with injections of Botox. Keep in mind that this can also just be a symptom of menopause, so for women it can be a new development after 50 that usually subsides within a few months to a few years.

Goosebumps. Those tiny bumps that appear all over your body from the cold or if you suddenly feel spooked, are a result of tiny muscles that connect the hair follicle with skin, which contract and make the hair stand on end. This an involuntary response associated with the fight-or-flight response and will regulate itself pretty quickly.

Shivers. Whether from cold weather or extreme emotions (such as shock), the shivers is a full body response that makes you feel chilled to the bone. You start to shake as an effort to bring the body back to a core temperature of 98.6°F. Even if its warm outside, wrap yourself in a blanket until it subsides.

Ringing in the ear. Known as tinnitus, ringing in the ear happens when you have fluid in your middle ear due to infection or congestion, or when you're chronically exposed to loud noises that can cause permanent damage. Protect your ears by earplugs when exposed to loud noises such as live concerts and professional sporting events — and don't be embarrassed to cover your ears with your hands when a loud train passes by, or if you're walking by a construction site.

Ear popping. When you experience a rapid change in altitude, the opening in your ear, known as the Eustachian tube, opens to release pressure, and you hear a pop. It can happen in a plane or even in a car when driving up and down in the mountains. This is the body's way of maintaining equilibrium. It will feel worse when flying or exercising at high elevation.

Twitching or tics in the eyes. These always seem to happen on exam days, or on important occasions when you want to look your best. That is because they are often a result of stress, tension, lack of sleep, extended staring, or eye strain. Sleeping well and reducing stress are key. Try closing your eyes and taking a few deep breaths, gently massaging or tapping around your eyes to get them to relax.

Seeing stars. If you stand up too quickly, get hit in the head, or have migraines, you may see stars as blood flow surges to different parts of your body. Last time I did a cartwheel across the floor it was like the 4th of July in my living room! While positional vertigo, or feeling dizzy upon standing up very suddenly, is fairly common — If you see stars for more than a few moments, you could have a tear in your retina and you should see your eye doctor immediately.

Yawning. It is almost impossible to hide, and we all associate yawning in public with being bored or sleep deprived. Tired or not, it is the body's way of regulating the amount of carbon dioxide and oxygen in your blood. Just be careful of yawning excessively while driving, as it is physically impossible to keep your eyes open when you yawn — not to mention that drowsy driving is extremely dangerous!

Hiccups. Hiccups are actually funny because the minute they start, everyone starts laughing. The diaphragm, which sits below the stomach, regulates our breathing. When we eat and drink too fast, or have a need to catch our breath, the diaphragm contracts and causes hiccups. You may also get hiccups in emotional situations or if your body experiences a sudden temperature change. In both of these cases, the hiccups are a result of a glitch in your nerve pathways, which is why a sudden scare can sometimes end an episode.

The only effective cure for hiccups is to tilt your head far forward and drink from the far side of a cup (don't turn the cup around, drink from the far side where it is). Somehow this affects the air in your throat and windpipe and puts an end to the session, no matter how long it has been going on.

Numbness in the arms and legs. Sitting directly on your feet or pressing your head on an arm or shoulder squeeze the nerves and sends a message to your brain to shut down. The sensation of pins and needles is the body re-awakening the nerves back to normal. This may happen while you sleep, especially if you are lying on your side or at an odd angle. As weird as it feels, it is totally harmless, and circulation returns to the area very quickly once you use it again.

Charley horse. These are muscle spasms or muscle cramps (usually in the calf) that happen so quickly you don't know what hit you. The best thing to do is get up and move around to help it subside. They are usually caused by dehydration, electrolyte imbalance, and strenuous exercise without proper nutrition. Sip water and orange juice to regain your fluid balance, and eat something with a bit of salt in it, but keep it healthy.

Cracking joints. It sounds like something is popping and cracking, and you may worry if you've hurt something — but this is just the sound of air being released from between the joints, like cracking your knuckles or getting a spinal adjustment. However, if you hear a popping sound accompanied by pain or swelling, you may have an injury that requires treatment. Get to know your body so you can tell the difference!

Burping. This occurs when the body is expelling excess air from your upper digestive tract. It is usually a result of swallowing air when you eat too fast, so it often happens during or after a meal. It can also occur when you are nervous and compulsively swallowing. Cover your mouth with your hand or a napkin and say, "Excuse me." You may wish to turn away from any company when breathing out after a burp in case your breath is bad. No need for embarrassment, though, everyone knows there's no way to stop a burp.

Farting. People often think they have too much gas in their system, or ate something that causes excessive farting, when in fact it is perfectly normal to fart all day long. Most people produce about 1 to 3 pints a day and pass gas about 14 to 23 times a day. Intestinal gas is made up of mostly odorless vapors, and the unpleasant odor of gas that we smell comes from bacteria in the large intestine that release small amounts of gases that contain sulfur.

If you are very uncomfortable, or suffer from painful gas buildup, it's a good idea to see a gastroenterologist and perhaps undergo some testing to isolate the problem. You may have to try an elimination diet to see if some particular food is causing the issue for you — don't just eliminate dairy or gluten or meat because those things are causing problems for your best friend, or because you read about it online!

Insomnia. We all have trouble falling asleep or staying asleep from time to time, but if this bothers you on a regular basis, it's worth discussing with a doctor. There are many practical things you can try to improve the quality of your sleep, including: (1) reducing your exposure to blue light, such as from computers, tablets, and cell phones, in the hours before bedtime; (2) making sure that there is no light in your bedroom, including light from alarm clocks, tv or cable boxes, and chargers; and (3) and trying various soothing sounds to lull you to sleep, such as soft music or various white noise machines.

All of these conditions may be annoying, but should not be a cause for grave concern. If they occur much more than you're comfortable with, on a daily or weekly basis, take notes on the frequency and severity of the occurrences, and discuss them with your doctor at your next checkup.

Interactive Chapter Review

Schedule a checkup, take notes on any conditions or concerns, and bring along a friend or family member to help you take notes on the doctor's advice.

*Which of these **Medical Specialists** have you visited:*

Internist/General Practitioner

Ear, Nose, and Throat specialist

Ophthalmologist

Dentist (Do you brush and floss every day? Remember, only floss the teeth you want to keep!)

Dermatologist (Do you use sunscreen every day, and avoid tanning?)

Gynecologist/Urologist

Gastroenterologist

Chiropractor

Orthopedist/Podiatrist

Physical Therapist

What steps have you taken to help prevent falls? Removed throw rugs, tidied up electrical extension cords, had hearing and vision tests, done balancing (proprioception) exercises?

*Do you worry about **Dementia and Alzheimer's**? Do you have a family member who suffers from these problems? Have you had any testing done to determine if you are a candidate for these conditions? Are you practicing prevention through mental and physical exercise to increase activity and blood flow to the brain?*

*Do you **sleep** through the night? If not are you willing to try techniques to improve your sleep?*

*Have you stopped **smoking**, or are you engaged in a smoking cessation program? How are you doing with that?*

*Have you reduced or eliminated **alcohol** consumption? Do you have a problem in cutting back? Do you find that you are drinking more than when you were younger? Can you find help if you need it?*

Do you experience more of any of the following conditions than you are comfortable with, on a daily or weekly basis? Can you seek help for these issues, or just learn not to be embarrassed or concerned when they arise?

Excessive itching

Excessive sweating

Ringing in the ear (tinnitus)

Goose bumps

Shivers

Charley horses

Numbness in the arms and legs

Burping

Farting

Yawning

Hiccups

Ear popping

Twitching/tics in the eyes

Seeing stars

Insomnia

Chapter 5
Eating Well

"Thou shouldst eat to live, not live to eat." – Socrates

Healthy eating means different things to different people. Let's dispel the myths about nutrition once and for all, and take a practical approach to eating well for life.

I came to appreciate the importance of eating well in early adulthood, and it was a giant step from how I grew up. For most of us born in the baby boom generation, our parents believed that eating was a means to stay alive, to pass on cultural traditions, or as a reward. Food was used to bribe children into behaving, and most of life's milestones were celebrated with food. Having an abundance of food represented wealth and prosperity. These beliefs are still prevalent today.

When the American population started to gain weight, and diseases related to obesity started to show up, health professionals took notice and started to put people on DIETS! From this point forward there was no turning back from the weight loss mania. Starting in the 1950s, providing people, especially women, with pills that revved up the metabolism was commonplace, and the cycle of taking pills, powders, and following wacky and sometimes dangerous food fads was in full swing.

"It is now more confusing than ever to understand what choices to make when managing our weight"

In my day-to-day work as a nutrition and fitness professional, I am constantly monitoring the bombardment of food and nutrition media hype that seems to come at us every day. If any of these fads really worked, we would all be in perfect shape. Many diets you see out now are recycled programs from years gone by, with a different name and a snazzy new package. We've finally moved from low fat being promoted as the key to weight loss, to eating clean by eliminating toxins and "Franken-foods" such as trans-fats, chemical additives and preservatives, and processed sugars.

Recently, we've heard more about diets that are high protein and high fat diets, like ketogenic, paleo, and Whole 30, which advocate cutting out most or all carbohydrates. This is a recirculation of ideas from years past, similar to low-carbohydrate or low-glycemic diets like Atkins or South beach. Keep in mind that all vegetables and fruits are carbohydrates! Beans are a combination of carbohydrates, protein and fat. Brown rice, whole grain bread and pasta, and sprouted wheat products are all carbohydrates as well.

"To eat is a necessity, but to eat intelligently is an art." – La Rochefoucauld

Realize that just by eliminating simple carbohydrates — candy, cookies, refined white bread, cake, soda, sweetened beverages and desserts — we are 90% of the way there. What is universal and shared by all healthy nutrition programs is the idea that if we eat foods closest to their natural state, with minimal processing, and no additives or artificial ingredients, we all would be a lot better off. The advent of fast food restaurants popping up everywhere since the early 1970s has made is very easy for us to get instant access to affordable food. Enjoy it once in a while, always being mindful of your food choices.

"Let food be thy medicine and medicine be thy food." – Hippocrates

Let's start with the basics and understand the composition of food:

Nutrients

A nutrient is a component of food that is needed to sustain life. Nutrients are divided into two categories based on the quantity needed by the body to function properly.

The first category is **macronutrients** — carbohydrates, proteins, and fats, which are required in larger amounts. The second category is **micronutrients** — vitamins and minerals which are required in smaller amounts. Water is the exception, it is considered a micronutrient, but the body requires a substantial amount of water every day.

Whether you are male or female, all of these nutrients are necessary to our survival, and must be present to provide energy, continued growth, and healthy functioning of the all of the body's processes. The proper balance of all of these nutrients can be fulfilled by eating a varied diet.

All foods yield energy, and a calorie is a measurement of that energy. The number of calories (heat released from energy) in a food product is determined by the energy provided in a gram of a macronutrient.

Carbohydrates have 4 calories per gram, protein has 4 calories per gram, and fat has 9 calories per gram. Micronutrients have no caloric value, but they all work together to sustain life.

> **"Typical American diets exceed the recommended intake levels or limits in four categories: calories from solid fats and added sugars; refined grains; sodium; and saturated fat." – USDA.gov**

Carbohydrates

These days the word "carbohydrate" seems to scare a lot of people. Carbohydrate gets its name from the composition of the molecule. It is comprised of carbon, oxygen, and hydrogen. All carbohydrates ultimately break down into the simple sugar glucose, to keep the energy and metabolism of the body steady. Carbohydrates are especially important for brain health. If the glucose levels in the blood stream dip too low, it can result in fatigue, fuzzy thinking and impaired cognitive function.

Complex carbohydrates, such as starchy vegetables, whole fruits, and whole grains, take longer to break down into the simple form, which is glucose, and thus have a slower rate of increasing blood sugar levels. **Simple carbohydrates**, such as white sugar, flour, refined rice, pasta, bread, cake, candy, soda, and yes, fruit juice, can drive up blood sugar almost immediately. This is why orange juice is used to revive someone who has fallen into insulin shock. Insulin shock refers to the body's reaction to too little sugar — hypoglycemia — often caused by too much insulin. Diabetic coma refers to a victim of high blood sugar — hyperglycemia — who becomes confused or unconscious.

When we eat too much carbohydrate, the body may not be able to metabolize the simple sugars fast enough, or thoroughly enough, to convert them into energy, so the sugar will stay in the blood stream and compromise other systems such as the kidneys and the heart. The body has a natural adaptation to store the excess sugars as fat, which can result in weight gain and insulin resistance and/or type 2 diabetes. (There are several types of diabetes, but we are just addressing diet-induced type 2 diabetes here).

Protein

Proteins are made up of carbon, hydrogen, and oxygen with a nitrogen molecule attached. Proteins are the basis for all metabolic processes in our bodies: muscle building, tissue regeneration and repair, hormone balance, blood clotting, and immune response, to name a few. Proteins are made from chains of amino acids and with 20 different amino acids in nature, our bodies have a remarkable ability to transform these chains into what we specifically need to stay alive. When we eat too much protein it will be stored as fat, which can lead to weight gain in the long run.

The main sources of **animal protein** are fish, poultry, meat, eggs, and dairy products including milk, cheese, and yogurt. You may also find **non-animal protein** in legumes such as soybeans, black beans, kidney beans, lentils, and other beans: a half cup of beans contains as much protein as one ounce of steak.

Eat Well Tip
Whole grains such amaranth, quinoa, and bulgur are very high in protein. Similar to rice, when combined with beans, they form a complete protein in the absence of animal products.

Ground nuts (peanuts and cashews) as well as **tree nuts** (almonds, hazelnuts, pecans, walnuts, macadamias) also contain protein. Recommended serving sizes for nuts are quite small: just a quarter cup has about 200 calories, so be careful about mindless munching or the calories add up fast.

There are 9 **essential amino acids**, and 11 non-essential. This means that the essential amino acids need to come from food, and the remaining ones are synthesized by the body as needed. It is very important if you choose to eliminate food groups from your diet, such as meat and dairy products, that you are balancing out the necessary requirements for your protein needs. This is why being vegetarian and vegan is of concern to many health professionals. They may not be condemning the practice, but it does make it more challenging to make sure your nutritional needs are met. When following a vegetarian diet, it is critical to be familiar with **food combining** in order to obtain all the needed amino acids for good health.

The best way to ensure that you are getting all of your necessary nutrients in a vegetarian diet is to combine rice and beans, corn and beans, quinoa, green leafy foods and soybeans. Nuts are also a good source of vegetarian protein, but try to mix it up so you are getting a variety of nutrients at all times.

Fats and Oils

Lipid is the chemical name for all fats and oils that occur in nature. Found in both plants and animals, fats are a very necessary nutrient. Fat is generally the term for fat substances that are solid at room temperature, and is of animal origin. Oils are defined as fats that are liquid at room temperature, and are derived from plants.

Triglycerides are the main constituents of fat in humans and other animals, as well as in vegetables.

Cholesterol, also necessary for health, is found mostly in animal fats, where plant fats do not have cholesterol. Cholesterol is a waxy, fat-like substance that's found in all the cells in your body. You need cholesterol to make hormones, vitamin D, and it is critical for helping you digest foods. Your body converts all the cholesterol it needs, where the excess can form plaque on your coronary arteries. The information keeps changing about what our cholesterol levels should be, and later on, I will discuss the levels and how to manage them.

Vitamins and Minerals

Although they are all considered micronutrients, vitamins and minerals differ in basic ways. Vitamins are organic and can be broken down by the environment inside and outside of the body. Minerals are inorganic and hold on to their chemical structure. *For our purposes here, organic means that the compound contains carbon, and inorganic does not.*

There are two types of vitamins: fat soluble and water soluble.

When you eat foods that contain **fat-soluble vitamins**, the vitamins are stored in the fat tissues in your body and in your liver. They wait around in your body fat until your body needs them. That is why they can be toxic in large doses. These are Vitamins A, D, E, and K.

Eat well tip
Healthy Fats — we hear a lot about including healthy fats in our food plan, but what is this really? Basically, it's avoiding saturated fats from animal products, and focusing on fats that are close to nature. So rather than relying solely on vegetable oils, eat fatty foods such as avocados, olives, and coconut. You can also obtain healthy fat in your diet from nuts and oily fish, such as sardines and salmon — but be careful about having too much fish, due to concerns about mercury and other contaminants in our oceans. Most of all, avoid fats when they are combined with sugars, such as in baked goods, dairy desserts like ice cream or sweetened yogurts, as the one-two punch of sugar and fat can be a killer.

The fat soluble vitamins help keep your eyes, skin, lungs, gastrointestinal tract, and nervous system in good working order.

Water-soluble vitamins don't get stored in your body. They are absorbed directly into the bloodstream, and are eliminated daily.

This group of vitamins includes Vitamin C and the B vitamins

> Thiamin - vitamin B1
> Riboflavin - vitamin B2
> Niacin - vitamin B3
> Pantothenic acid - vitamin B5
> Vitamin B6
> Biotin - vitamin B7
> Folic acid (folate), B9 Vitamin B12

Although water-soluble vitamins have many tasks in the body, one of the most important is helping to free the energy found in the food you eat. Water-soluble vitamins should be replenished every few days.

No matter how well we eat, it is almost impossible to have the full complement of vitamins without supplementation. A general multi-vitamin is good for everyone, and you may wish to increase your dose of certain vitamins or minerals to address specific issues. Consult your doctor, pharmacist, or natural health food store to discuss which supplements would benefit you in particular.

Minerals

Minerals are categorized as **major minerals** and **trace minerals**. They are all essential for our health and well-being, but are necessary in varying quantities.

Major minerals travel through the body in various ways. Potassium, for example, is quickly absorbed into the bloodstream, where it circulates freely and is excreted by the kidneys, much like a water-soluble vitamin. Calcium is more like a fat-soluble vitamin because it requires a carrier for absorption and transport.

> Sodium
> Chloride
> Potassium

Calcium
Phosphorus
Magnesium
Sulfur

Major minerals are necessary to balance the water in the body. The ratio of Sodium, Chloride, and Potassium are key in fluid balance and cardio-vascular wellness. Calcium, Phosphorus, and Magnesium are instrumental in keeping our bones healthy. Sulfur helps stabilize protein structures, including some of those that make up hair, skin, and nails.

Along with exercise as an adult, building strong bones before the age of 30 is the best defense against developing osteoporosis in later years. Adults above 19 years old should be consuming at least 1,000 milligrams of Calcium per day. Women can lose up to 20 percent of their bone mass in the five to seven years after menopause, and men can experience bone density loss as a result of a drop in testosterone with age.

Table salt is a compound of Sodium and Chloride. Ingesting excess sodium in the body causes it to bind to calcium, and both will be excreted when the body senses that sodium levels in the bloodstream are too high. This causes us to lose much-needed calcium, which may lead to or worsen osteoporosis, and also forces the kidneys and urinary tract to work harder. This is another reason why reducing our sodium intake through salt and processed foods is recommended.

Trace minerals are found in extremely small quantities in the body, yet their contributions are just as essential as those of major minerals such as calcium and phosphorus, which each account for more than a pound of your body weight.

Iron
Fluoride
Zinc
Copper
Chromium
Iodine
Manganese

Molybdenum
Selenium

Trace minerals carry out a diverse set of tasks. Here are a few examples:

Iron helps carry oxygen throughout the body

Fluoride strengthens bones and wards off tooth decay

Zinc helps blood to clot, is essential for taste and smell, and bolsters the immune response

Copper helps with iron absorption and the formation of hemoglobin, which carries oxygen in the blood

Trace minerals interact with one another, sometimes in ways that can trigger imbalances. The difference between "just enough" and "too much" of the trace minerals is often tiny. Generally, food is a safe source of trace minerals, but if you take supplements, it's important to make sure you're not exceeding necessary levels.

Antioxidants

We hear a lot about Antioxidants, but what are they? Antioxidants protect cells from damage to DNA, cell membranes, and general wear and tear on the body that comes from normal metabolism. They are synthesized in the body as needed, as well as naturally occurring in the color pigments of fruits, vegetables, beans, nuts and seeds. That's precisely why eating a plate full of mixed fruits and vegetables is very sound advice!

Your body can self-regulate because cells naturally produce plenty of antioxidants to help protect them, but you can help the process by wisely choosing the foods you eat and supplements you take.

Here are a few examples of antioxidants, many of which you are probably already getting in your diet: **Carotenoids** from lycopene in bright red tomatoes, and lutein in dark green kale. **Flavonoids** like anthocyanins in purple blueberries and grapes, quercetin in apples and onions, and catechins in green tea. **Vitamin C** and **Vitamin E** and the mineral **Selenium** also have antioxidant properties.

Eating a colorful diet is the best way to get your antioxidants. Think of a rainbow, and choose your items accordingly.

Water

Water is the source of life. 60 percent of our bodies are comprised of water, as well as 90 percent of the bloodstream. The benefits are obvious but it is always good to review. Water is good for your joints, saliva and mucous membranes, is great for good skin and hair, cushions the brain and spinal cord, regulates body temperature, improves digestion, and is necessary to maintain a good metabolism.

As noted above, even though water is considered a trace mineral, you still need an abundance of it for good health. There are many different opinions on how much water you should be drinking every day. Coffee, tea, juice and soda all contribute to hydration but water is the best source, so make it your go to beverage when thirsty. We have all heard that eight to ten 8-ounce glasses a day is the way to go. Why not, it will not hurt you and most certainly will help you. Hydrate!

Eat a Variety of Nutritious Foods from All Food Groups

Pay attention to the food that you consume each day. You may be eating plenty of food, but your body may not be getting the nutrients it needs to be healthy. Nutrient-rich foods have vitamins, minerals, fiber and other nutrients but are lower in calories. To get the nutrients you need, the staples in your diet should be primarily vegetables and low-sugar fruits such as berries, melons, and grapefruit, and some moderate-sugar fruits including apples, peaches, pears and oranges.

Vegetables and fruit are high in vitamins, minerals and fiber — and they're low in calories. Eating a variety of brightly colored produce may help you control your weight, cholesterol, blood pressure, and overall reduction of body fat.

Color is essential when eating a healthy diet. You will get the best benefit from your vegetables and fruits by eating a variety of them every day. The richer the color, the higher the levels of phytonutrients. The color pigment is where the nutritional value lies. Green leaves, yellow, orange and red vegetables and fruits, bean varieties, and citrus fruits are all great sources with a high nutritional value that you can consume every day.

Unrefined whole-grain foods contain fiber, and that can help lower your blood cholesterol and help you feel full, which may help you manage your weight. Beans are a great source of both fiber and protein as a standalone, or in the absence of meat. Eating large amounts of high-fat foods adds excess calories, which can lead to weight gain and obesity. Emphasize fats from healthier sources, such as eggs, low fat cheeses, vegetable oils, nuts, olives, and dairy products.

Eat fish at least twice a week. Recent research shows that eating oily fish containing omega-3 fatty acids may help lower your risk of death from coronary artery disease. Examples of oily fish include salmon, trout, tuna, swordfish, mackerel, herring, sardines and anchovies.

If you drink alcohol, drink in moderation. That means one drink per day, preferably when you are in for the night so you stay safe.

Artificial Sweeteners

Chances are you have eaten something with an artificial sweetener in it today. Once used mostly for replacing sugar in your coffee or slashing calories in soda, artificial sweeteners are found in almost every type of packaged foods. Can these sugar substitutes really help you slim down? Some studies seem to indicate that simply

Preparing Nutritious Food

Many households are very busy in the morning with preparing to go to work, getting kids off to school, maybe having older family members living with you that also need attention. The best way to solve this is have an evening routine that sets you up for success in the morning. Have everything you need to start your day, ready to go the night before, so there is no scrambling when you need to leave.

Eating at night is considered bad for you because as a rule, you will be sedentary for the rest of the evening. However, in reality, your body burns calories all day just for baseline functioning, so the time of day is less important, and the quality of food is of utmost importance. Managing your nutrition schedule is best accomplished by following your own signals of hunger, thirst, and a general sense of when eating feels best for you.

The number one problem that most people face each day is not being prepared to eat healthy, and thus we end up eating whatever is around the house, or ordering out. Do your best to have healthy choices on hand so even in the most hectic of situations, there is always something to eat! Many people like to do meal preparation over the weekend for the week ahead, planning shopping lists, meals and menus to suit their nutritional goals.

There is so much information and misinformation about when and how to eat, and I stand by the old adage, breakfast is the most important meal of the day — a healthy breakfast, that is. No real meal plan for the morning results in skipping this most important meal, or running to the drive-through or grabbing a donut at work.

As noted above, you don't need to cut out food groups, or be strict about following a 3-meals-a-day plan, or having many small meals throughout the day, or fasting part of the day. At some point you need to get at least 1200–1500 calories a day into your body for baseline metabolic functioning.

Eat well tip
Break the Soda Habit! Try some of the many new flavored sparkling waters, either unsweetened or with natural non-caloric sweeteners such as stevia or monk fruit. Make your own infused waters in your fridge, with cucumber slices, lemon, oranges, or strawberries. Treat yourself every day as if you were at the spa!

having a sweet taste — even with no calories behind it — can trigger an insulin response.

Worse still, often when we use artificial sweeteners, we're overly optimistic about how many calories we're saving and often end up eating more than we should. A common example is having that big piece of chocolate layer cake, with a diet soda or black coffee with an artificial sweetener. For the long term, a good goal is to try and retrain your taste buds to eat less sugar and sugar substitutes.

Tracking Your Food

One thing that every person does who has successfully lost and kept off a lot of weight is to track and monitor their food. In the past this was done with notebooks and food diaries; now you can find a dozen apps online that make it easy to look up food calories and track what you eat, from meat and fish, to fruits and vegetables, to nuts and dairy products. They often have calorie counts and nutrition information for restaurant meals as well.

Check out *Spark People, My Fitness Pal, Lose It!* and other online food/exercise trackers to see which one works for you. Most have a free version you can use, as well as paid versions with more bells and whistles.

As much as possible, it's a good idea to make your own meals at home. That way we know what's going into what we eat, no mystery ingredients, extra fat, salt or sugar, etc. You can select organic fruits, vegetables, meat, milk, poultry, and eggs. You can add your own spices and herbs. Even a simple roast chicken from the store can have brown sugar in the glaze! Always check the ingredients.

When you do your own food preparation, you can use food labels as a guide to help determine just how many grams of each nutrient a given food item provides. Even if a particular food is seemingly high in calories, it can still be good for you. Eating a well- balanced diet shouldn't be a battle between junk and health food. It is a lifelong approach to making good choices throughout the day, the week, and the month, that will make a difference over the course of a lifetime.

What we look for in the calorie count is the grams of carbohydrate, protein, and fat. For each nutrient, multiply the number of grams by the calories per gram to get the percentage of each item from the total calories — keep in mind there are 4 calories per gram of carbohydrates, 4 calories per gram of protein, and 9 calories per gram of fat.

Nutrition Facts

8 servings per container

Serving size   **1 (84g)**

Amount per serving

Calories   **103**

	% Daily Value*
Total Fat 3g	**4%**
Saturated Fat 0.5g	**3%**
Trans Fat 0g	
Cholesterol 0mg	**0%**
Sodium 50mg	**2%**
Total Carbohydrate 12g	**5%**
Dietary Fiber 2g	**6%**
Total Sugars 6g	
Includes 0g Added Sugars	**0%**
Protein 7g	
Vitamin D 0mcg	0%
Calcium 83mg	6%
Iron 0.9mg	4%
Potassium 70mg	2%

* The % Daily Values (DV) tells you how much a nutrient in a serving contributes to a daily diet. 2000 calories a day is used for general nutrition advice.

So in this example, that means there are 48 calories of carbohydrates per serving (4 x 12) and 28 calories of protein (4 x 7), plus 27 calories of fat (9 x 3) for a total of 103 calories (48 + 28 + 27 = 103) as shown on the label. It is also important to note that there are 0 trans fats in this product, and less than one-third of the total calories come from fat.

Learning how to make better food choices and adopting an overall healthy lifestyle is a process. It takes time to realize that you have no reason to eat at fast food restaurants, you don't have to eat food you don't like, and you have every right to say no to bad food even if it means disappointing family and friends — there is no need to be polite at the expense of your own health.

"Savoring the good in every day is what living well and aging well is all about. Good food and drink, with good company, will always have a lasting impact on your overall well-being. 'Food, glorious food,' as it is celebrated in the musical 'Oliver!'"

Basal Metabolic Rate (BMR)

As noted in the previous chapter, when you embark on the journey of getting healthier, is always a good idea to get a wellness assessment of your overall body from a doctor, fitness professional, nutritionist, or chiropractor.

One of the things that they may advise — or help you to do — is to learn your individual **Basal Metabolic Rate** to be sure that you are using up at least as many calories as you take in. Get to know how many calories you should be eating and drinking to maintain your weight — then subtract just 500-1000 calories per day from your maintenance figure. That results in a calorie deficit per week of 3500-7000 — the safe weight-loss amount of 1-2 pounds per week!

A quick way to calculate your Basal Metabolic Rate (BMR) is an equation known as the Harris-Benedict Formula:

Women
BMR = 655 + (4.35 x weight in pounds) + (4.7 x height in inches) - (4.7 x age in years)

Men
MR = 66 + (6.23 x weight in pounds) + (12.7 x height in inches) - (6.8 x age in years)

Take the time to do this calculation — it will result in more calories than you think! But be sure to use one of those food trackers so that you don't eat more calories than you know you can burn up every day... and remember to reduce the total calorie goal by

500-1000 calories per day if you want to safely lose 1-2 pounds per week.

> ## "If we could give each individual the right amount of nourishment and exercise, not too little and not too much, we would have the safest way to health." – Hippocrates

Body Mass Index (BMI)

Another important figure to know is your Body Mass Index (BMI). You can find online calculators for this, and tables as well, such as the one below. There is a broad range of "healthy" weights at each height — and very muscular bodies tend to weigh more. This is a good general guideline for what works for each of us.

Body Mass Index

	WEIGHT																									
HEIGHT	120	130	140	150	160	170	180	190	200	210	220	230	240	250	260	270	280	290	300	310	320	330	340	360	380	400
5'0"	23	25	27	29	31	33	35	37	39	41	43	45	47	49	51	53	55	57	59	61	63	65	66	70	74	78
5'1"	23	25	27	28	30	32	34	36	38	40	42	44	45	47	49	51	53	55	57	59	61	62	64	68	71	75
5'2"	22	24	26	27	29	31	33	35	37	38	40	42	44	46	48	49	51	53	55	57	59	60	62	65	69	73
5'3"	21	23	25	27	28	30	32	34	36	37	39	41	43	44	46	48	50	51	53	55	57	59	60	63	67	70
5'4"	21	22	24	26	28	29	31	33	34	36	38	40	41	43	45	46	48	50	52	53	55	57	58	61	65	68
5'5"	20	22	23	25	27	28	30	32	33	35	37	38	40	42	43	45	47	48	50	52	53	55	56	60	63	67
5'6"	19	21	23	24	26	27	29	31	32	34	36	37	39	40	42	44	45	47	49	50	52	53	55	58	61	64
5'7"	19	20	22	24	25	27	28	30	31	33	35	36	38	39	41	42	44	46	47	49	50	52	53	56	60	63
5'8"	18	20	21	23	24	26	27	29	30	32	34	35	37	38	40	41	43	44	46	47	49	50	52	55	58	61
5'9"	18	19	21	22	24	25	27	28	30	31	33	34	36	37	38	40	41	43	44	46	47	49	50	53	56	59
5'10"	17	19	20	22	23	24	26	27	29	30	32	33	35	36	37	39	40	42	43	45	46	47	49	52	55	57
5'11"	17	18	20	21	22	24	25	27	28	29	31	32	34	35	36	38	39	41	42	43	45	46	47	50	53	56
6'0"	16	18	19	20	22	23	24	26	27	29	30	31	33	34	35	37	38	39	41	42	43	45	46	49	52	54
6'1"	16	17	19	20	21	22	24	25	26	28	29	30	32	33	34	36	37	38	40	41	42	44	45	48	50	53
6'2"	15	17	18	19	21	22	23	24	26	27	28	30	31	32	33	35	36	37	39	40	41	42	44	46	49	51
6'3"	15	16	18	19	20	21	23	24	25	26	28	29	30	31	33	34	35	36	38	39	40	41	43	45	48	50
6'4"	15	16	17	18	20	21	22	23	24	26	27	28	29	30	32	33	34	35	37	38	39	40	41	44	46	49
6'5"	14	15	17	18	19	20	21	23	24	25	26	27	29	30	31	32	33	34	36	37	38	39	40	43	45	47
6'6"	14	15	16	17	19	20	21	22	23	24	25	27	28	29	30	31	32	34	35	36	37	38	39	42	44	46
6'7"	14	15	16	17	18	19	20	21	23	24	25	26	27	28	29	30	32	33	34	35	36	37	38	41	43	45
6'8"	13	14	15	17	18	19	20	21	22	23	24	25	26	28	29	30	31	32	33	34	35	36	37	39	42	44
6'9"	13	14	15	16	17	18	19	20	21	23	24	25	26	27	28	29	30	31	32	33	34	35	36	39	41	43
6'10"	13	14	15	16	17	18	19	20	21	22	23	24	25	26	27	28	29	30	32	34	35	35	38	40	42

Underweight: BMI = less than 18.5

Normal weight: BMI = 18.5 to 24.9

Overweight: BMI = 25 to 29.9

Obesity Class I: BMI = 30 to 34.9

Obesity Class II: BMI = 35 to 39.9

Extreme Obesity: BMI = 40 and above

Most important of all, don't be depressed or disheartened if you're in the "overweight" or "obese" area — one step at a time can move you from one category to the next. And best of all: just making better food choices and getting more active will improve your health, even if your weight doesn't seem to budge.

What Works?

I am a huge advocate of Weight Watchers because the system works. You don't cut out any one food group, they provide recipes and food charts to work with, and best of all, the support groups are fantastic. You can lose weight, socialize, make new friends, date, and do it all in a healthy environment. Having other people around with the same focus and goals will help you to succeed. Taking charge of your health is a club you want to be part of! The lifetime support feature ensures that this is truly a lifestyle change, not just a fad diet.

Another program that has a lot of success is Overeaters Anonymous, based on the 12 steps of recovery. This support group focuses on the emotions of unhealthy eating and really helps individuals who have a problem with food or dieting in any area of their life: compulsive overeating, under-eating, food addiction, anorexia, bulimia, binge eating, or compulsive exercising. Again, the support feature helps you to stay connected and focused, rather than just try a quick fix to lose weight.

Many people have had success following a wide range of different programs, including low-fat diets such as Pritikin, low-carb/high-fat (LCHF) programs such as Atkins or Keto, or variations on that such as Sugar Busters, Paleo, or Whole 30. Another approach is Intermittent Fasting (IF), where you wait 12-16 hours to break your fast, or fast on a regular basis (interestingly, this has also been shown to increase longevity), using meal replacement shakes to reduce calories and increase protein absorption. You can also try a volume-based diet, where you select foods that have low caloric density (usually high water-content foods such as vegetables) so you eat a large volume of food without increasing calorie intake.

While personally I do not advocate cutting out any food groups or using meal replacements, I realize that everyone is individual in this regard, and different approaches may work better for some people. Find out what works best for you and your lifestyle, and what you can maintain going forward in your family and community. What matters most is consistency and persistence; whatever program you select, be sure it's one you can stick with for life.

Any healthy food program that you choose to follow will say the same thing: No fast food, no junk food, no sodas or sugary drinks, no fried food, and no processed food. As noted before, this will get us 90% of the way there. Many will also suggest limiting or eliminating "white" food, such as white sugar, white rice, white flour, and all of their associated products (pancakes, pasta, cookies, cakes, pies, sugar-sweetened ice cream, soda, candy, etc.). Once you start to limit these items in your diet, you should see a major difference in the way you feel... and in how your clothes start to fit.

Health professionals recommend weight loss for obvious reasons, but the methods by which you attempt to achieve it should be to improve your health, not make you sick. Trying some crazy fad diet where you just eat cabbage soup or cleanse with lemon juice and red pepper can leave you hungrier and sicker than when you started — and more likely to gain back any weight that you do lose. When you approach weight loss as a means of lowering cholesterol, blood pressure and risk of disease, everything else is a fringe benefit.

Be careful not to cut back too drastically on calorie intake, or your body will respond by conserving energy, reducing your basal metabolic rate and making those extra pounds harder to shed. As you improve your food choices, increase your activity level so that you will continue to burn calories, even at rest.

Increase Activity to Burn More Calories

Increase the amount and intensity of your physical activity to match (or exceed) the number of calories you take in. Aim for at least 30-60 minutes of moderate physical activity on most days of the week or — best of all — at least 30 minutes every day. Weight training ("lifting") in particular can help you to build muscle that will burn calories even while you're at rest. The next chapter will provide more detailed information on how to achieve this goal.

In general, regular physical activity can help you maintain your weight, keep off weight that you lose, and help you reach physical and cardiovascular fitness, which will also improve your mood, attitude, and outlook on life. If you can't do at least 30 minutes at one time, you can break it up into two 15-minute sessions, or three 10-minute sessions throughout the day. Remember the active folks who live in the Blue Zones (detailed in Chapter 1), where physical activity is part of their everyday lives! Start incorporating movement into your day-to-day routine.

"You cannot exercise your way out of a poor diet." - Anonymous

Nowadays everything is so automatic, we don't move. We use remote controls for the TV, automatic switches to start the car, talk to Siri or Alexa to turn on the lights, and sit at our desks to go shopping. We also tend to surround ourselves with food and make every social activity a food-based one. Try making a date to meet a friend for a walk in the park rather than at a coffee shop or restaurant. Being more active and getting sufficient sleep will also help you to make better food choices and manage your weight naturally.

But don't think that climbing a flight of stairs means you can eat two cookies! You'd be amazed at how few calories walking or running actually burns off, it is not enough to offset a fast-food binge or even a second helping. Mostly, exercise is good for the heart and lungs, as well as your mind and mood. That it can help to manage weight is just a positive side-effect. Remember: "You cannot exercise your way out of a poor diet."

Age-related Weight Gain

"Middle-age spread" is a derogatory term that describes the very dangerous form of weight gain that is common as we age. Fat tends to accumulate more readily in the abdominal area, which increases your risk of all common diseases. There are no quick fixes on this one. Eat healthy and exercise within your capabilities and you will see progress.

As we age, both men and women over 50 tend to move and exercise less than their younger counterparts, which can lead to weight gain. The number of calories you need for energy decreases as you age because aging promotes the replacement of muscle with fat. Muscle burns more calories than fat does. When your body composition shifts to more fat and less muscle, your metabolism slows down. (This is why lifting weights and building muscle can be so beneficial in controlling weight as we age — again, more on this in the next chapter on fitness.)

Genetic factors may play a role in weight gain as well. If your parents and other close relatives carry extra weight around the abdomen, you may be predisposed to do so, too.

Adult-onset weight gain can also have serious implications for your health. Excess weight increases your risk of high cholesterol, high blood pressure, and insulin resistance, which can lead to type 2 diabetes. These combination of risk factors also put you at increased risk of heart disease, stroke, and dementia. Many of the ailments that afflict older people are exacerbated by excess weight, such as arthritis, fatigue snoring, sleep apnea and COPD.

There's no magic way to avoid weight gain as you get older. The strategies for maintaining a healthy weight at any age remain the same: reduce your stress, monitor your hormones, maintain your blood sugar levels, and get sufficient sleep.

Gaining weight after menopause can increase a woman's risk heart disease and cancer. Obesity has been linked to an increased risk of developing breast cancer shown by many scientific studies. There is evidence to suggest that excess body fat at the time of breast cancer diagnosis is associated with higher rates of cancer recurrence and death. Furthermore, studies have shown that obese women are more likely to have large tumors, greater lymph node involvement, and poorer breast cancer prognosis with 30% higher risk of mortality.

Women who lose weight after menopause can reduce their risk of breast cancer by that much and more. Even small amounts of weight loss after menopause lead to a modest risk reduction.

Same goes for men. The risk for all diseases from heart problems, lung insufficiencies and all male cancers can be dramatically reduced with weight loss, improved diet, and exercise.

For every 10 extra pounds above a healthy weight that you have on your body, you increase your risk of obesity related diseases such as diabetes and heart problems. So, what you can do nutritionally to prevent or reverse age-related weight gain?

Be aware that your metabolism will naturally slow down as you get older. You need about 200 fewer calories a day to maintain your weight as you get into your mid- to late 40s and beyond. This shouldn't be a problem if you eat only when hungry and only enough to satisfy your hunger. You can also offset this change if you increase your activity levels, which can rev up your metabolism — maybe not back to what it was when you were 20 or 30, but much more than if you remain sedentary.

Most people gain weight as they age because the metabolism slows down, and they become less active — but they keep eating the same as they did when they were younger. If you cannot train or inspire yourself to eat less and move more on your own, consider joining a program that will help you to do so. It may save your life!

Interactive Chapter Review

What does "Healthy Eating" mean to you? Take a few minutes and think about what you think of as healthy eating.

How closely to you adhere to what you think of as a "healthy eating" plan? Have you given up trying to follow a particular program because every few years it seems there's a new "healthy" approach? What could make you decide to try once more?

Have you started to cut back on sugar, flour, fried foods, processed food, sugary drinks? What could help you to do so?

*Do you understand the importance of the various **nutrients** in food? What are the calorie counts for carbohydrates, proteins, and fats? If you're a vegan or vegetarian are you careful to track your food combining to be sure you are getting complete proteins?*

Do you take **vitamin** and **mineral** supplements? Have you checked with your doctor, pharmacist or health food store to see if there are particular supplements that would benefit you?

What colorful vegetables do you enjoy and include in your food plan on a regular basis? Which ones could you try that you don't use right now? Do you enjoy the lower-sugar fruits, and other fruit in moderation? Can you avoid sugar and artificial sweeteners?

Have you started **tracking** your food? What system or app do you use? Are you consistent — and honest — in tracking everything you eat?

Do you prepare most of your meals at home, or read labels and menus carefully when eating out to be sure you avoid sugar, salt, fat, and flour?

What techniques have you used to resist foods you know are bad for you, when they're pushed on you by well-meaning family and friends for "special occasions" or if you're at an event?

Take the time to calculate your **Basal Metabolic Rate (BMR)**, and your **Body Mass Index (BMI)**, and use these to guide your plan — and track your progress.

Have you tried group programs like Weight Watchers or Overeaters Anonymous? Do you benefit from the group support? What about following another formulated eating plan, low-fat, low-glycemic, low-carb, or something else? What works for you?

Have you begun to increase your cardiovascular activity to burn more calories? What about doing weight training to raise your metabolic rate so you continue to burn calories even at rest?

Chapter 6
Fitness

Why Exercise?

Health professionals the world over have fallen short in their attempts to get the majority of the population to embrace a fitness lifestyle. Why is that? It just seems too hard for most people. Fitness should be a fun, easy, and happy part of our day, but instead it seems like an extra chore or a burden that is added on to an already overwhelming schedule which leaves us exhausted every day.

> **"To restore life to your life, to defeat aging, to regain the youth you still possess, get your body in motion." – George A. Sheehan**

The number one motivator that drives me to exercise almost every day is my family. I don't ever want to be a burden on them, and I know that even the minimal amount of daily movement will stave off the ill effects of a sedentary lifestyle. Second, the thrill I get from my everyday accomplishments are enhanced when I exercise. I reduce my stress, I feel energized to tackle the days challenges, and I sleep better. Last but not least, if I keep up with my fitness regimen on a regular basis, I can afford a day off once in a while without any health setbacks. It is a like a bank account where I can make deposits and live off the interest in a down period.

> **"When it comes to healthy aging, all roads lead to movement"**

This chapter provides advice on both small and big changes we can make on a daily basis to incorporate fitness into your life. The best benefit from exercise, any kind, is that it invigorates us even when we are tired. I am always pleasantly surprised to experience an elevation in my mood when I exercise, even when I am very tired. That's a feeling I can really embrace, and everyone benefits.

Act Your Age

How old I look is important to me. Physicians, however, primarily concern themselves with biological age. How old are the arteries? The kidneys? The heart? Those questions run through a doctor's mind when faced with a patient who looks older than expected.

In my practice, I have seen many people whose lifestyles accelerated their biological aging. Our optimal life span is a little over 100 years — some say 120. But we begin quite early in life to diminish our longevity and ultimately settle for less. Blame part of this loss on our gene pools. Some people come from short-lived stock susceptible to the major killers: heart disease, diabetes and cancer. Some are vulnerable to artery disease and high blood pressure. These people must be very diligent in order to maintain their normal biological ages.

We also have a physiological age, measured by our physical fitness. If you didn't know your chronological age, how old would you be? Surprisingly, the average American is 30 years older functionally than he or she is chronologically. An active 60-year-old and an inactive 30-year-old will have equal physical work capacity.

At one time, physiologists thought people aged functionally from 10-15 percent a decade. Now we know this is far from the truth. Fit individuals show about a five percent loss in endurance per decade. The distance world records for the 40 age group fall within 5 percent of actual world records. At age 50, they come within 10 percent. At age 60, they are close to 15 percent.

These statistics clearly show that apparent aging can be blamed largely on inactivity. Inactive people give aging →

a bad name. People think it is normal to look, perform and have the arteries of a person 20 to 30 years older. When they see a truly normal individual, they typically remark how young he or she looks.

Yet, we can all stay young. We can all hold the aging process at bay. Many individuals prove we can remain lithe and supple. Loss of flexibility says we are old even when we feel young inside. That's why yoga and range-of-motion exercises should become our best friends.

Keeping our arteries young is a life-long task. We must not accept the generosity of medical advisors who allow us to weigh more and have higher cholesterol because we've grown too old for it to matter. It always matters. Cardiologist Paul Dudley White, pioneering fitness advocate of the 1950's, said we should not gain a pound after age 25. And, I would add, we shouldn't gain a milligram of blood cholesterol, either.

Among these undertakings, we can maintain youthful performance the easiest of all. We can forget whatever ravages time has done and simply put our bodies into action. With use, our bodies grow young. And over time we can regain the physiological losses we have incurred by sitting around on our duffs. "Life is motion," said Aristotle. To restore life to your life, to defeat aging, to regain the youth you still possess, get your body in motion.

There you have it. A prescription to make your chronological, biological, and physiological ages coincide. When that occurs, you may find that other people your age view you as an oddity.

'Why don't you act your age?' they will ask.
And you can reply, 'I am.'

Keep in mind that in order to move forward with your wellness goals, you may need to leave some old habits behind. Giving up certain behaviors and attitudes to reclaim our health can be very scary. But there is some good news: There is a misconception that you must run a marathon, win a dance competition, be as strong as a bodybuilder, as thin as a fashion model, or as flexible as a yoga instructor, to gain any benefit from your fitness activities. This couldn't be further from the truth. Any movement, any effort towards wellness is great for your body, mind, and spirit, and will improve the quality of your life.

"Exercise is king. Nutrition is queen. Put them together and you've got a kingdom" – Jack LaLanne

My personal heroes, Jack LaLanne and Joe Weider, were tireless in their advocacy for fitness throughout the human lifespan, promoting physical activity and good nutrition for all. They both lived to a very advanced age, and their programs and approaches are still used today, keeping fitness at the forefront for healthy aging. I love Jack Lalanne's saying, "Exercise is king. Nutrition is queen. Put them together and you've got a kingdom."

While being fit to obtain aesthetic results is important to a lot of people — in reality, the ideal body that many strive for is pretty close to impossible to achieve. Having these kinds of unrealistic goals can add to your stress load, as you work out more and more trying to mold your body into something that simply is unattainable... and then feel depressed and fall off the "fitness wagon" when you don't reach those sought-after results.

Often we find, especially with age, that no matter how much we exercise, we cannot lose weight. Weight loss is a multi-faceted process which requires extreme diligence in what we eat and how we live our lives, and should not be the sole goal of fitness. Regardless of what you weigh, the physical benefit of exercise is plain and simple, stronger bodies fare better when aging then de-conditioned bodies. Love your body as it is, and maintain your health.

"Lack of activity destroys the good condition of every human being, while movement and methodical physical exercise save it and preserve it." - Plato

Benefits of Fitness

Whether you are a long term fitness enthusiast, just starting out, or somewhere in between, exercise is essential to keeping your cardiovascular system in tip-top shape, and enhancing your brain function. With age, your risk increases for all diseases — yet a good strong heart and healthy lungs can stave off those risks, as well as the physical decline we associate with aging, for many years to come. Being active is the perfect complement to healthful, energizing foods. If you keep up with both exercise and nutrition, the results will follow.

Being physically fit is obviously important for our physical health, and the positive impact on our brains is phenomenal. The brain functions to keep our bodies adaptable, and guides us in carrying out many complex processes at once. When the brain continues to be nurtured and challenged, we stay highly functional at a much older age than our sedentary counterparts.

"It is a shame for a man to grow old without seeing the beauty and strength of which his body is capable." - Socrates

In your 40's and certainly on to your 50's, you will start to see the signs of cardiovascular and muscular decline. Don't panic! You can always strengthen your body at any age with the proper type and amount of exercise.

A strong heart pumps more oxygenated blood throughout the body with fewer heartbeats. This reduces the wear and tear on the cardiovascular system as a whole. Regular exercise also helps keep cholesterol levels down, regulates blood pressure, and enhances your ability to keep your nervous system in check. Even a small amount of daily physical activity helps strengthen your lungs, and improves endurance, so you can tackle longer intervals

Sobering Statistics
According to the Physical Activity Council:

• Only one in three children are physically active every day, spending more than 7.5 hours per day in front of a screen (TV, videogames, computer, tablet, cellphone)

• Less than 5% of adults participate in 30 minutes of physical activity each day, and only one in three adults receives the recommended amount of physical activity each week

• Only 25-34% of adults 65-75, and 35-44% of adults 75 years or older are physically active

• Only one in five homes have parks or fitness centers within a half-mile

While there have been steady year over year increases in physical activity from 2013 to 2018 — even so, during that time period over a quarter of the entire American population ages 6 and up reported no physical activity whatsoever. In 2018, 82.1 million people did nothing, ignoring established findings that a regular fitness routine will "boost stamina and focus throughout the workday, encourage healthier eating habits, reduce poor coping skills (such as drinking alcohol and eating processed and sugary foods), and reinforce these habits with children." (Physical Activity Council)

of exercise, giving you better circulation and more energy for your day to day living.

Don't Regret the Past — Just Start Now!

You can start exercising now, and whatever your physical limitations are, there is always room to improve. As one yoga master put it, "You're never too old, never too bad, never too late and never too sick to start from the scratch once again." There is no added benefit to becoming a ninja warrior. Just a desire to enjoy life more on a daily basis can be enough motivation to be the best you can be at any age. The three areas that we focus on for improving our physical and mental well-being are **aerobic activity** for cardiovascular health, weight and resistance **training** for strong muscles, and **alignment and balancing** movements to maintain our symmetry, flexibility, and functionality for years to come. Later in the chapter, I will discuss chair fitness for those of you with limited mobility.

"The first wealth is health." – Emerson

Aerobic Activity/Cardiovascular Exercise

Let's start with a simple exercise that improves overall heath with very little effort: walking. Walking incorporates cardiovascular fitness, endurance, weight bearing exercise, and improves balance. I have now made it my primary form of daily exercise, and add other workouts in where I can.

Walking is often perceived as a moderate form of exercise that doesn't do much. Contrary to popular belief, walking has all the benefits that you can derive from swimming, running, and biking.

Gat a pair of good athletic shoes and you are off! Whether indoors or out on the street, I find that it is ideal way to see the world and spend time with friends and family. There is no right or wrong way to do this, walk for you and you alone.

If your goal is to maintain your weight, or reverse the results of a bad lab report, start with walking on the treadmill at home, or hitting the streets for some external stimulation. Like all forms of exercise, walking will boost your mood and improve cognitive function.

To monitor my progress, I wear a step counter and strive to walk a minimum of 10,000 steps a day. Instead of being married to a number, just keep at it and have fun.

For the more competitive among us you can start off walking and work your way up to running. There is no shortage of road races that you can walk and run, with distances spanning from 5ks which is 3.1 miles up to marathons at 26.2 miles and beyond!!

Meet up with a friend to ensure you show up for your daily walk. Many people get a dog to ensure they get out once a day! Enjoy being out in nature when the weather is nice, and take shelter in a local gymnasium or mall when the weather is rough. You will find mall walking groups in many communities.

Strength/Resistance Training

The next component of fitness that keeps us strong and upright as we age is resistance training. You can achieve this by working out with weights, or using your own body weight. Challenging your body to push against gravity outside of your comfort zone has amazing results. For those of you who feel comfortable around a gym, get back in there and get started. Even using light weights and building up as you go will get you stronger.

If you are new to weight training, it might be worth investing in a trainer or group classes that will be manageable for you. Many gyms now offer the Silver Sneakers program . This is a series of fitness classes geared toward the older adult to improve fitness without the risk of injury. Their website, www.silversneakers.com, will steer you to a local facility that holds these classes. Even better, if you are on Medicare and have supplemental insurance, they will pay in full.

Balance/Stability (Proprioception)

Lastly, and in my opinion, the most important factor in staying well as we age, is maintaining balance and keeping the body stable. You will inevitably have challenges with your stability, and exercises that counter this are the best way to go. As we age, our sense of balance is compromised due to loss of muscle and bone mass, and our senses that keep our bodies aware of our surroundings start to diminish. Particularly, our sight and proprioception (this is how our body senses gravity and body placement while moving).

Maintaining balance is easy and will help keep you stay injury free while engaging in all the activities of daily living as they relate to balance. The best programs for balance are yoga, Tai Chi, and all the martial arts. For a quick pick me up first thing in the morning, 10 toe touches really help.

Stretching/Flexibility

With each passing decade, your muscles and tendons are less elastic and there is an increased risk of tearing or spraining tissue and breaking bones. It is perfectly okay to continue to exercise rigorously, but it is equally important to rest and stretch in between. If you exercise every day, alternate high impact activity such as running and weight training, with low impact activities such as yoga, stretching and leisurely walks. If needed, take one day a week off to fully recover, and get a good night's sleep so your body can heal.

Functional Fitness

A practical application of staying fit as we age is functionality. This is where you will apply your fitness to the practical applications we use in our daily lives.

Strong arms and back let you lift and carry items without being hurt. Stretching and flexibility comes in handy when you need to reach up high into a cabinet to retrieve something, or bend down and twist to reach something under a chair — or an airplane seat. Good balance helps you to resist and avoid falls that can be catastrophic as we age.

"Leave all the afternoon for exercise and recreation, which are as necessary as reading. I will rather say more necessary because health is worth more than learning." – Thomas Jefferson

Healthy heart and lungs from regular cardiovascular exercise will enable you to go up and down stairs as needed, have endurance for long days, enjoy vacation travel, and best of all, running and playing with your grandchildren — or your other healthy adult friends!

Staying independent as long as possible makes you have a better quality of life every day. No one wants to be infirmed and dependent on others for day to day needs of living.

Recreational Exercise

At the very least, engage in recreational exercise. This should be fun and can be free if you look for ways to enjoy the outdoors on your own or with friends. Go for a hike or a walk in the park — or at the local shopping center! You know that daily aerobic exercise burns calories and strengthens the heart and lungs, resistance training staves off muscle loss and strengthens bones to prevent frailty in later years, and stretching improves flexibility.

But most important is to be active on a daily basis. Thousands of people buy new gym memberships on January 1st, and then never go! Sometimes investing in a personal trainer or joining a running club is worth it if it makes you actually show up and work out.

But if you're bored or pressured by repetitive, "meaningless" exercise, try something different: how about a Zumba class, water aerobics, swimming, square dancing, belly dancing, flamenco, skiing, snowboarding, rowing, kayaking, canoeing, rollerblading, surfing, hot yoga? You could join a local club sports team, and play volleyball, softball, basketball, flag football, soccer, tennis, badminton, even ping pong or bowling. Try Pilates, Barre classes, boxing, jazzercize, martial arts (including judo, tae kwon do, karate, capoeira, aikido and others), spin class or road biking or trail biking or mountain biking! Get a "class pass" that lets you try out different modalities and providers in your area to see which works for you. Find something you love to do, and you will be more inclined to keep up with it.

If you don't automatically love something, try reading books about people who have achieved goals in various sports, and see if their mental tips and tricks could work for you. Many people say, "Oh, I hate running, it's so boring" – but then when they learn techniques to stay engaged and improve, it becomes a fascinating activity, a great way to learn and grow and meet other health-focused people.

"If you are embarking on a new sport or activity that you haven't tried before, learn proper techniques from the experts, and vary your activities to avoid repetitive stress injuries"

Tips for Persistence and Motivation

Following these simple tips will help improve your staying power when it comes to keeping up your fitness. First off, before you start any exercise, warm up properly by moving and dynamic stretching. Even on days when you don't have hard exercise planned, it's a good idea to stretch your muscles to stay loose and flexible.

Try to space your workouts evenly throughout the week. Saving all of your physical activity for the weekend is more likely to end up in injury and excessive soreness which will increase your chances even more of getting hurt — that's why they call people who do that "weekend warriors." If you are embarking on a new sport or activity that you haven't tried before, learn proper techniques from the experts, and vary your activities to avoid repetitive stress injuries.

Sometimes when we start something new, our enthusiasm gets in the way of our safety. Don't overdo mileage or speed, and take a day off between challenging workouts to allow muscles to recover. Increase the intensity of the activity slowly, and when you are used to it, you can take on a more challenging level.

"When starting any new program, just focus on the first step"

On any day when your motivation is flagging, try a few simple tips to get out the door and get moving:

> Lower your goals for the day — perhaps you have too demanding a training schedule. If need be, tell yourself it's okay to do an easier run or workout than you had planned.

Eat or drink something to rev up your engine — not a lot, just a tiny bit to get going.

Tell yourself, "I'm just going for a walk," put on sneakers and head out the door — then throw in a few running steps, or head to the gym, and before you know it, you're enjoying an energetic workout!

Smile, and know that you are doing something good for yourself!

"Exercise and temperance can preserve something of our early strength even in old age." – Cicero

Olympian Jeff Galloway is one of the great experts on motivation for exercise, and on the positive effects of being active (particularly running and walking) on your brain chemistry, and thus improving your mental state. He talks and writes at length about strategies to get motivated and stay motivated, how to get around the logical left brain telling you that you can't do something and tap into the creative right brain that helps you achieve the impossible. Galloway provides insight about vision, magic words, and dirty tricks to help you achieve your goals. He also discusses the importance of getting checked out to make sure there's nothing physically or medically wrong that is interfering with your performance or ability. For tips on how to get moving when you're unmotivated, check out www.jeffgalloway.com or one of his many books on running and walking.

"To keep the body in good health is a duty... otherwise we shall not be able to keep our mind strong and clear." – Buddha

Determining Your Fitness Level

It is critical to determine your current fitness level, and know where you really are right now, because this will play a role in how you plan to stay strong and flexible as you age.

Plan Out your Exercise

Write out a schedule for your exercise and stick to it. i.e., go to the gym Monday and Wednesday, run on Tuesday and Thursday, do Yoga on the weekend — or whatever works for you. Spin class, dance lessons, tennis matches — having a consistent plan every day, and keeping it the same from week to week, will help you stick with it.

Again, preparing the night before will ensure success in the morning: lay out your workout gear, so you can hop right into your clothes when your bed is calling you for just five more minutes. Prepare any drinks or snacks you like to have during or right after your workout. Schedule your workouts into your calendar, the same way you would any other appointment, and don't let anything interrupt your plan. If someone asks you to go out at a time that you'd planned to go for a run or get to spin class, just say, "I'm sorry, I have an appointment at that time, can we get together later?" or "Unfortunately I'm otherwise engaged, let's plan on another time." You don't have to explain that you're exercising, that's your business.

Committing to your fitness, and devoting time to prepare for it the night before, makes it far more likely that you will be consistent in your workouts. Before you know it, you will be a regular exerciser!

Here is a tried and true fitness test that I have been using for many years to help people assess their fitness level, particularly in relation to their chronological age. This fitness test was devised by Wayne Wescott, PhD, of the South Shore YMCA in Quincy, Massachusetts. Wayne is the author of *Get Stronger, Feel Younger.*

Below are 5 tests to determine your current level of strength, core, flexibility, balance, and cardio-vascular fitness, and where each one of these should fall in relation to your age.

Wherever you fall on the scale, you can always work to improve so that everyday tasks will not become more difficult with age. Once you have determined your level, you can do these exercises 2–3 times a week to dramatically improve all aspects of your wellness.

Strength

Strong muscles make you more capable of functioning physically, and they boost your metabolism, helping your body to burn calories even when at rest.

Dips Test. Sit on a very sturdy chair or bench and slide your body off, while gripping the front edge with both hands to support yourself. Make sure your arms are and legs are straight, then bend your elbows to a 90° angle, and press back up. Repeat as many times as you can, and stop at 15.

Repetitions	Body age Correlation
13-15	20's
10-12	30's
8-9	40's
5-7	50's
3-4	60+

Core

The core muscles in your abdomen, back, and hips hold you upright and allow the upper body and lower body to work together. Having a strong core will prevent back problems as you age.

Bicycle Test. Lie on your back, with your knees over your hips, feet dangling in the air. Place your hands behind your head and try to touch your right elbow to your left knee as you fully straighten your right leg. Return to the center without touching your shoulders to the floor. Switch sides and try to touch your left elbow to your right knee. Repeat. Count until you can't go any further, it you get to 20, you are finished.

Repetitions	Body age Correlation
17-20	20's
13-16	30's
10-12	40's
8-9	50's
5-7	60+

Flexibility

Flexible muscles and joints help you maneuver better in the world. Getting stiff can set you up for injury, and if you reach beyond your range you risk getting a strain.

Reach Test. Sit on the floor with your right leg straight in front with the foot flexed. Place your left foot against your inner thigh, with the left knee open to the side. See how far you can reach towards the toes of your foot.

If your hand doesn't reach your toes, measure it as a negative distance, i.e. -2 inches. If you reach your toes it's 0, and if you can pass your toes it's +2.

Inches	Body age Correlation
3	20's
2	30's
1	40's
0	50's
-1 or less	60+

Proprioception (Balance)

In order to stay upright and walk with certainty into your 80's and beyond, you must work on your balance. An alarming number of deaths occur due to falls that are a result of people losing their balance.

One Leg Balance Test. Stand near a wall or chair in case you need support. Balance on your right leg, resting your left foot on your right calf. With a clock or a timer, see how long you can hold that position, with your eyes closed. If that is too challenging, start with your eyes open.

Seconds	Body age Correlation
16-20	20's
14-15	30's
12-13	40's
10-11	50's
8-9	60+

Cardiovascular Endurance

When your cardiovascular system is healthy, blood carries oxygen to your muscles as needed. Therefore, you shouldn't be winded climbing a flight of stairs or running for the bus. This can be improved at any age, but if the heart and lungs are compromised it can be difficult to perform the easiest of tasks.

Step Test. Using a curb or stairs, step up and down for a total of 3 minutes. Stop and take your pulse, counting for 15 seconds. Multiply by 4 to find your beats per minute. The idea is to increase your cardiovascular fitness, which results in a lower heart rate per minute, making the body more efficient at rest.

Beats per minute	Body age Correlation
105-107	20's
108-110	30's
111-113	40's
114-116	50's
117+	60+

Make it your goal to be active for a total of 30 minutes or more a day on most days. Increased physical activity, including strength training, may be the single most important factor for maintaining a healthy body composition — more lean muscle mass and less body fat — as you get older.

"An apple a day keeps the doctor away" - Proverb

Seated Workouts

Even those who are wheelchair bound, injured, or very infirm and unable to stand, can benefit from seated upper body workouts. Sitting up tall in the chair ensures you engage your abdominal muscles to maintain good posture.

Warmups include **Seated Punches**, forward, to the side, and up in the air, and **Shoulder Retractions**, where you extend your arms then pull them back bent at the elbow. Workouts can use equipment, like balls, bands, or dumbbells:

Eat well tip
Always have something to eat before a workout, a hard-boiled egg, a handful of almonds, or an apple will do. Drink water as you go, it is easy to get dehydrated, even with minimal effort.

If you do more strenuous or lengthy exercise, such as endurance running, you will want to carry nutrition and hydration with you, and refuel along the way, such as gels, sport beans, or sports drinks.

After a long workout, you want to have protein as soon as possible for the muscles to rebuild. A protein shake, chocolate milk (including almond or cashew milk if you are lactose intolerant), or some cooked chicken are all good choices.

Medicine ball exchange. Hold a small weighted ball in one hand to the side, then pass it overhead into the other hand, and lower the arm down to the other side. Repeat.

Medicine ball chest press. Hold the ball in both hands in front of your chest, then extend your arms until elbows are almost straight, then bring it back.

Chest press with band. Wrap a TheraBand around the back of your chair, hold each end in your hands, and extend your arms forward.

Overhead press with alternating arms. Hold dumbbells in each hand, press weights straight overhead and then lower back down; then alternate one hand and then the other.

Front raise with triceps extension. Hold the dumbbells out in front of you, raise them overhead with straight arms, then bend your elbows to drop the weights behind your head.

These and many more exercises may be found online, at websites such as www.verywellfit.com and www.vivehealth.com.

"Exercise is a journey, not a destination"

Chair Yoga

Even the benefits of yoga are available to those who are unable to be weight-bearing, whether due to age, infirmity, or injury. Yoga is noted for helping reduce stress, pain, and fatigue, as well as improving joint lubrication, balance, and flexibility. Here are several seated yoga poses anyone can try. To start, sit firmly in the chair, towards the forward edge but still stable.

Seated mountain (Tadasana). Sit up straight, extend your spine, root down into the chair with the base of your sit bones, take a deep breath and roll your shoulders down your back. Pull your belly button in toward your spine, and relax your arms down at your sides. Engage your legs by lifting your toes and pressing firmly down onto the ground with all edges ("four corners") of your feet.

Warrior I (Virbadrasana I). Start in Seated Mountain, take a breath, lift your arms out to your sides until they meet overhead. Interlace fingers, keeping pointer fingers and thumbs out to point at ceiling, for more intensity try to bring your palms together to touch. As you exhale, roll shoulders away from ears and let shoulder blades slide down the back. Relax and take 5 deep breaths in this position before releasing clasped hands on an exhale and let arms float gently back to your sides.

Seated Forward Bend (Paschimottanasana). Start in Seated Mountain, focusing on extending your spine, and simply fold forward over your legs. You can start with hands resting on your things for extra support, or keep them at your sides. Take 5 or more breaths in this pose, which massages your intestines to help digestion, as well as lengthening spine and stretching back muscles. When ready, inhale and lift back to an upright position, using your core to pull yourself up.

Eagle Arms (Garudasana). Take a breath, stretch your arms out to the sides, then as you exhale swing them together in front of you, right arm under left, and grab the opposite shoulder with your hands to give yourself a hug. To increase flexibility, rotate your hands and wrap forearms around each other until your right fingers are in your left palm (perhaps they're just grabbing the base of the thumb). Inhale and lift your elbows, exhale and roll down your shoulders to relax them away from your ears. Take a few breaths, repeating elbow lift and shoulder roll if desired, then relax.

Reverse Arm Hold. Inhale, stretch arms out to sides, palms down. Exhale, roll shoulders forward, bend elbows, and clasp hands behind your back, holding on to whatever you can reach (fingers, hand, wrist, elbow), gently pull hands apart without releasing the grip. Take 5 slow, even breaths, then switch the grip, and release gently on an exhale.

Simple Seated Spine Twist (Parivartta Sukhasana). Twisting poses help with lower back pain, digestion, and circulation. They also feel great! Remember that although you have the chair back to help you twist, don't yank yourself farther than you can turn naturally; forcing a twist can cause injury. Inhale, extend your spine, raise arms to the sides; exhale, gently twist to one side with upper body and lower your arms — one hand on top of the chair back, one resting at your side. Look over your shoulder and use your grip to help you stay in the twist but not to deepen it. Hold the pose for 5 breaths, release and repeat on the other side.

Single-leg stretch (Janu Sirasana). Move toward the edge of the chair, but don't slide off! Sit up tall, stretch out one leg to rest the heel on the floor, toes pointing up. Rest both hands on outstretched leg, inhale, straighten your spine, then exhale and bend over outstretched leg, sliding your hands down your leg. Take the stretch as far as you like without straining or forcing anything and still feeling supported by both chair and your hands. Inhale and exhale slowly and evenly 5 times in this position, gently going deeper; repeat on the other side.

It's very common for one side to be more flexible than the other, don't be surprised if this is true in your case in any of the above exercises.

Interactive Chapter Review

Why Exercise? How are you doing as far as adopting a fitness lifestyle? Do you still regard fitness as a chore, something you "have" to do — or have you started to see it as something fun, something you "get" to do?

Do you still think you have to be super-fit to get any benefit from exercise? Or have you started to see that you can start small?

Are you still attached to the idea that working out is just to look a certain way, achieve a specific body type or weight goal? Or have you begun to develop health and fitness goals that are not attached to an aesthetic ideal?

Benefits of Fitness. What other benefits have you seen — or do you hope to see — from a fitness lifestyle? Improved mood and attitude? Brain functioning? Physical strength? Flexibility? Better balance and agility? Not huffing and puffing when you have to climb the stairs or run for a bus? Being able to play with your grandchildren — or active adult friends?

Do you feel you're too old to start now? Do you still regret that you didn't start when you were younger, or that you gave up fitness levels you had achieved years ago? What can you do to motivate yourself and jump-start a new program today?

What **cardiovascular** activities have you tried? Walking? Running? Rowing? Biking? Skiing? Dance? Do you use a step counter or GPS watch to track how far you walk each day?

How about **strength** training? Have you tried weightlifting, or doing body weight exercises such as pushups, dips, and squats to build muscle?

Do you follow any programs to improve your **balance** and **flexibility**? What are they?

What aspects of **functional fitness** do you need to focus on? Do you have trouble climbing stairs or walking fast to cross the street? How about lifting heavy bags, or reaching into a high cabinet? Can you twist and bend down if you drop something?

Recreational Exercise. What kind of exercise do you like to do for fun? Do you like team sports, like basketball or softball or bowling? Or more solitary pursuits, such as weight training, running, walking, hiking, biking, or skiing (all of which you can also do with others, if you enjoy the company)?

How successful are you at being active on a daily basis? What would help you to do so? Have you tried out different activities to see what you like and what you'll be able to do consistently?

Have you read and practiced different approaches to help you be more **motivated and persistent** in your pursuit of fitness? What tips and tricks do you use when your motivation is flagging? It's important to have a personal approach that works for you.

Have you done the **fitness test** to determine your current fitness level? Write down your results with the date, so you can see how you improve as you go forward! Note down your levels of Strength (dips test), Core (bicycle test), Flexibility (reach test), Balance (one leg balance test), and Cardiovascular Endurance (step test).

*Have you made a **personal goal** to be active at least 30 minutes a day on most days? Do you realize this is the best way to prevent age-related disease and loss of function? Have you tried seated workouts and/or chair yoga, for those days when you're just too tired to go out (or perhaps you're nursing an injury)? These are great ways to remain active even if you can't be weight-bearing at the current time.*

*Do you **schedule** your exercise for the week, so you know what you're doing each day? How about laying out your needed clothes and supplies the night before, so you're more likely to work out in the morning and be consistent with your exercise routine?*

*Have you planned in your **rest and recovery** from your exercise by focusing on how to improve your sleep schedule? Do you suffer from insomnia? What have you done to address this? Reducing evening screen time? Covering up light sources in the bedroom? Trying various soothing sounds or music? Natural supplements? Have you noticed that you are sleeping better since you are exercising more?*

*Have you set clear, written, daily **goals** for yourself? Do you benefit from reading a daily meditation guide? Do you use an exercise journal, or meal planner, to track practical aspects of your day? How about putting yourself and your health goals first — have you started to say "no" to things that interfere with your fitness schedule? Have you put your workouts and classes on your calendar as appointments you must keep?*

Chapter 7
Appearance As We Age

Personal Appearance As We Age Is Very Personal!!

Visible signs of aging appear much earlier than most of us may want to acknowledge. For women this is often more difficult to accept because society can be so unforgiving. Men get away with a bit more until a certain age, but then both men and women must struggle for acceptance as their appearance indicates their advancing years.

Just a few of the things we encounter along the aging highway: Unwanted facial hair, hair on your head turning white or gray, thinning hair, balding spouses (both men and women), sagging skin, and changes in our body type (expanding waistlines and widow's hump). All of this can be a natural part of aging, and yet we all can't help but feel shocked when it happens to us. These are some of the realities of aging that all the exercise and healthy food in the world won't change.

"64% of workers have seen or experienced age discrimination in the workplace." − EEOC

It is very helpful, and very freeing, to fully acknowledge your age. Accepting your age, and accepting your current appearance, brings you into the present and helps you move forward. I have noticed the difference in time, money, and concern spent about hair upkeep between those who decide to color their hair and have to have regular root touch-ups, and those who decide to "go gray." I still color my hair the same brownish-black that I have been my whole life. My family and friends all tell me they don't see me as a person with gray hair. I often wonder if it's the fear of one's own mortality that keeps me and others from allowing nature to take its course. Many friends of mine have just decided to go gray and I love the way they look. Whichever way you choose to go, you are the only one that needs to feel comfortable with your decision.

Certain aspects of self-care become more important as we age, especially hair removal: men have to trim ragged hairs on their

Gray hair is synonymous with aging — the new lingo when referring to our population aging is the "Graying of America," "The Silver Tsunami," and the Medicare-endorsed fitness classes for the 65-plus are called "Silver Sneakers." The truth is that gray hair can appear at any time throughout one's lifetime, with some people starting to go gray as early as their teens. There is a movement now to express ourselves as we are, gray hair and all!

Historically, men with gray hair are considered experienced and distinguished, the silver fox, yet when women appear in public with gray hair, they are considered unkempt, past their prime, "letting themselves go," or not attractive anymore.

So much has changed, yet many of us are still stuck in the old ideas that equate an aging appearance with a diminished ability to contribute to society. As children, we were taught to refer to the women with gray hair as the "old lady," and gray-haired ladies in movies were always the grandma or the evil witch.

Let's work together to dispel those antiquated ideas, embrace the idea that going gray is natural, and you can look fabulous at any age!

eyebrows, nose, ears and neck, and women may have to spend more time or money on depilatories, plucking, electrolysis, waxing, or laser hair removal — excess facial hair is one of the "markers" of aging that is easy to control. On the other hand, some women have less body hair on their legs or underarms than when they were younger, reducing the need for frequent shaving, waxing or depilatories.

"Having your own sense of style is very personal. If you dress appropriately for your body type — which has nothing to do with age — you will feel much better about yourself"

Do not let your perceived appearance of yourself stop you from living life to the fullest. Especially when it comes to having relationships, old and new. As we age, you will find that people really have learned that it's what's inside that counts, and not to judge a book by its cover. There is a plastic surgeon on every corner, but keep in mind that nipping and tucking will not make up for unhealthy choices in terms of exercise and nutrition. Having your own sense of style is very personal. If you dress appropriately for your body type — which has nothing to do with age — you will feel much better about yourself.

A few examples of ways to maintain a more positive frame of mind regarding our appearance as age:

Let go of worrying about how you look in a swimsuit, just focus on the water and how good it is for you to swim. Enjoy the freedom of floating and moving in the water. Besides, once you're in the water, nothing else matters!

Be grateful for your health and well-being to remain active and engaged in life, many are not so fortunate. My favorite story about maintaining a positive attitude: when asked how it felt to be confined to a wheelchair, the older man responded, "I am not confined by my wheelchair, I am liberated by it. Without the wheelchair I would be bed-bound and unable to get out and explore the world around me." There's always a positive way to regard our situation, and turn perceived limitations into benefits.

Keep in mind that wearing your glasses, hearing aids, and orthotics in your shoes, are not limitations — they are all ways to keep yourself safe and able to enjoy life and those around you.

Remember that while you may not look as young and fresh as you did in your teens or 20s, you have experience and knowledge that you sorely lacked in those days. Draw upon that to maintain your confidence.

You're old enough to know that those who judge you by your appearance, and write you off because you're "too old," are superficial and not worth your time — and they're the ones missing out on all you have to offer.

Ignore articles about "what to wear at 40" or "best haircut at 50" – if you want to wear a bikini, or long hair, or a mini skirt, and feel comfortable doing so — do it. The body positive movement has given us great freedom to enjoy life just as we are, so if you want a "beach body" – just take your body to the beach!

Don't try to compete with younger people in terms of physical appearance or athletic prowess — let them enjoy their time in the sun. Know that you have your own standards of beauty and fitness, and you are comfortable in your own skin.

"If you want a beach body, just take your body to the beach!"

Tips on Feeling Good at Any Age

Dress well every day. Why wait for a special occasion to feel special? Get rid of any clothes that make you feel old, fat or unattractive. Don't even wear them around the house when no one is looking. Dress each day in a way that makes you feel good about you. Work hard to feel attractive for yourself, not for your partner, or the outside world.

If you feel it's necessary, get a makeover, including hair, manicure, pedicure, facial or professional makeup session. For maintenance, treat yourself to one of these salon services regularly (at least once or twice a month). Not in your budget? Have a ladies' pamper party, where you get together with friends and share your skills, do a deep hair condition, use facial sheets, polish each other's nails. It's a great way to build closer connections, so important as we age.

Men can enjoy self-care treatments as well: I often see men getting a manicure/pedicure, and everyone enjoys a good massage or facial. Many spas and vacation settings offer "couples massages" or other treatments. As they say, moisturizing is good for anyone with skin!

"Some of the worst mistakes in my life were haircuts." – Jim Morrison

Address any medical conditions or physical issues that may prevent you from leading a full, rich life. Visit your doctor, take your vitamins or prescribed medications, do your exercises and physical therapy — whatever you need to do to live at your best. You will be able to do more things that you love, and you may even inspire others to improve their own self-care as you model good behavior.

Of course, read through the previous two chapters about eating energizing, healthful food, becoming more active in your daily life, and finding fun sports or other physical activities that improve your circulation and brings color to your cheeks. Taking care of yourself makes you feel better than ever, and that will show in how you carry yourself, from your smile to your posture to your stride.

"We are truly lit from within"

And just like our bodies, our minds and memories can slow down as we age. Mental games are a fun way to keep your brain fit and active. Meaningful work or hobbies give you a vibrancy and energy that others can see, enhancing your beauty from the inside out. No matter what we look like, there's nothing as wonderful as someone who makes you think of the Billy Joel song title, and loves you "*Just the way you are.*"

One of my favorite activities to do with my family is play Scrabble. It's a long-standing tradition from my childhood, that has carried over with my siblings and our children. We have so much fun, and laugh the whole way through! The energy and excitement you project when you talk about or share your interests — whether doing needlepoint, or surfing the waves — lights up your face and helps you connect with others in a new way. We are truly lit from within.

"Being the best version of you is just being yourself"

What Can You Do To Achieve Your Personal Best?

Realize that you cannot change your basic body type, and try not to compare yourself to others. You are who you are, and no one else can be you!

That said, you can certainly work to be the best you can be — if you've never been active before, look at examples of other people who became active later in life. You'll be amazed at how many people never started walking, running, or swimming, or dancing, until their 40s or 50s or even older — and have come to love their new activities, which add youth to their years. It's never too late to find something you love to do — or decide to love something you know will benefit you.

"None are so old as those who have outlived enthusiasm." – Henry David Thoreau

Invest time and money in yourself in ways that make you feel your best. Examples include: getting a massage, buying new workout clothes or fitness equipment (like walking shoes, gym bag, resistance bands, free weights, etc.), enrolling in a yoga, dance, or martial arts class, going to a spa retreat, sports camp, or yoga vacation. Avoid spending money on diet products, "anti-aging" creams, and other items you know are a waste, designed and marketed to help slim your wallet, not your waistline or your eye bags.

Weighing yourself regularly may be a valuable guideline, but only do so (at most) once a week, and be sure to choose the same time of day and wear the same amount of clothes each time. It's normal for weight to fluctuate by a couple of pounds (up or down) daily or even at different times in the same day, due to fluid shifts or how much you eat and drink throughout the day. Weighing yourself every day will drive you crazy, and not really provide any useful information on how you are progressing or maintaining your weight.

Perspiration and eliminating your waste also plays a role in weight maintenance and overall health. Just about any exercise program, along with most diets, will provide some initial benefit as far as weight loss — though at first it may just be as a result of losing "water weight" through these methods. Persistence and consistency will lead to results over the long run — results that you can live with as your lifestyle truly changes.

Fashion For Life

Dressing well for your age doesn't translate into buying expensive clothes or throwing out everything you own. Young people dress in what is known as cheap chic — we did the same thing in years past, shopping in army-navy stores or secondhand shops (now called "vintage"). That is not how you want to look 20 years into your adulthood and beyond. Find a style, a "look" that works for who you are today.

"Following trends is futile, next thing you know you're out of style"

Note that this doesn't mean you are relegated to baggy clothes that hide your body. Find clothes that flatter your figure and make you feel good — that will get you further than trying to look like your teenager, or even how YOU looked as a teenager! Just because all the rage is a sideways baseball cap, doesn't mean you should give up your personal style in an effort to blend into a crowd you probably won't feel you belong in anyway.

Everyone has a personal style. I try to take the time to spend a weekend afternoon in my closet. I take out every article of clothing I own and try it on. I make sure it is during the day, in the sunlight, in front of a full-length mirror. I ask my daughter and my husband what they think and I then can get an honest critique. Clothing store dressing rooms have very flattering mirrors and lights. How many times have you bought something, love the outfit in the store and hate it when you get home? Return these items or donate them if they are old. There is no need to hold on anymore, let them bring joy to someone else.

Do your undergarments fit properly? A professional bra fitting is priceless. Go to a store and get help from the staff about what styles work for your body today. It takes out the guesswork and you will feel a lot better when you stop wearing too tight underwear. When shopping for these items, I ask for the most senior salesperson working in the store, they are usually the most helpful.

Are your clothes frayed and stained? Do you have old t-shirts and sweatshirts that remind you of a rock concert from 25 years ago, but are no longer wearable? Throw them out now! It is another step in the direction of freeing yourself from the past, especially any painful parts of your history. However, if these clothes commemorate something you love and want to remember, cut them into squares to make a memory quilt — or just take a photo with your phone and create an electronic collage. When my parents died, rather than keeping large items I couldn't use, I have their keychains and luggage tags that I use on a regular basis. Less clutter, same memories!

"The average American woman owns 30 outfits — one for every day of the month. In 1930, that figure was nine." - Forbes

Clean out your clothing closet — reduce your inventory. Follow the 80/20 rule: You probably wear 20% of your clothes 80% of the time. I know I do. Only keep what you absolutely love. It is cheaper in the long run. As a recovering clothes horse, I go shopping a lot less often because I have a minimal amount of clothes that I wear all the time. I only go out and buy something new when I absolutely need it.

Like many of us, of all ages, I keep a lot of black clothes in the closet — because I think black makes me look thinner. Try to have some color in your wardrobe to brighten up your day!!! Even if black pants or a little black dress is the order of the day, add a touch of color with a bright top, jacket, or scarf to add some interest. Brightly colored shoes or a purse can also spark up your look.

Fashion Tips for Adults:

Clothing that fits right for you. Too-tight clothing is never flattering and usually too revealing — but too-baggy clothes can make you look sloppy and even bigger. Buy clothes to fit the fullest parts of your body, and find a good tailor to nip in the rest.

As for style, while it's easy to stay with what has worked for you over the years, now might be a time to try a new look: if you've always worn tailored, fitted clothes, experiment with a flowy, bohemian look — and vice versa. You may discover something new that you love, and that works for your body and personality today.

> **"Always keep in mind that you and only you decide where to live, how to dress and how to live for optimal happiness"**

Perfume or cologne. Apply scents very sparingly. If you spritz too much by accident, put some rubbing alcohol on a cotton ball and dab off the excess. Rather than spray the cologne on yourself, spray it in the air and walk through it! If you've always liked florals, perhaps try something woodsy or peppery or citrusy for a change, and vice versa.

Be aware that it can be extremely offensive to others when you are drenched in perfume, and rather than say anything, most people will just avoid you, and probably not tell you why. If traveling or dining with friends, make sure they do not have high scent sensitivity — some people cannot tolerate fragrance of any kind.

"In Praise of Older Women" – Frank Kaiser, Suddenlysenior.com

One of the perks of dufferdom is an increased capacity to appreciate people. Friends. Spouses. And, for me, women. All women. When I was 20, I had eyes only for girls my age. Any woman over 30 was ancient, over 40 invisible. Today, at 65, I still appreciate the 20-year-old for her youthful looks, vigor, and (occasional) sweet innocence. But I equally enjoy women of my own age and beyond, and every age in between. I've learned that each has its own special wonders, attractions, magic and beauty.

As I grow in age, I value older women most of all. Here are just a few of the reasons senior men sing the praises of older women:

An older woman will never wake you in the middle of the night to ask, "What are you thinking?" An older woman doesn't care what you think.

An older woman knows herself well enough to be assured in who she is, what she is, what she wants, and from whom. By the age of 50, few women are wishy-washy. About anything. Thank God!

An older woman looks great wearing bright red lipstick even in glaring sunlight. This is not true of younger women or drag queens. And yes, once you get past a wrinkle or two, an older woman is far sexier than her younger counterpart!

Her libido's stronger. Her fear of pregnancy gone. Her appreciation of experienced lovemaking is honed and reciprocal. And she's lived long enough to know how to please a man in ways her daughter could never dream of. (Young men, you have something to look forward to!)

Older women are forthright and honest. They'll tell you right off that you are a jerk if you're acting like one. A young →

---

woman will say nothing, caring what you might think of her. An older woman doesn't give a damn.

An older, single woman usually has had her fill of "meaningful relationships" and "commitment." Can't relate? Can't commit? She could care less. The last thing she needs in her life is another dopey, clingy, whiny, dependent lover!

Older women are dignified. They seldom contemplate having a screaming match with you at the opera or in the middle of an expensive restaurant. Of course, if you deserve it, they won't hesitate to shoot you if they think they can get away with it.

Most older women cook well. They care about cleanliness. They're generous with praise, often undeserved.

An older woman has the self-assurance to introduce you to her women friends. A young woman with a man often will ignore even her best friend because she doesn't trust the guy with other women. The older woman couldn't care less.

Women get psychic as they age. You never have to confess your sins to an older woman. They always just know.

Yes, we geezers praise older women for a multitude of reasons. These are but a few. Unfortunately, it's not reciprocal. For every stunning, smart, well-coifed babe of 70 there's a bald, paunchy relic in yellow pants making a fool of himself with some 22-year-old waitress.

Ladies, I apologize for us. That men are genetically inferior is no secret. Count your blessings that they die off at a far younger age, leaving you the best part of your lives to enjoy and appreciate the exquisite woman you've become. Without the distraction of some demanding old fart clinging and whining his way into your serenity.

Revealing skin. In a professional capacity, showing too much leg (or chest/décolletage) is never a good move — for women or men. Revealing a little skin makes men appear overly casual or sloppy, and for women, it may be an attempt to look more sexy, but in reality, you may not be taken seriously.

In a casual setting, such as a party or family event, you can be more relaxed, but covering up is always a good idea, especially when it comes to cleavage — the sensitive skin in this area is one of the first parts of the body to show age.

However, all bets are off at the beach and the pool, where you should enjoy the freedom of not having to be clothed — though as noted above, it can't hurt to seek out a swimsuit that suits your body type. A plunging neckline or high-cut derriere or teeny tiny bikini might have been flattering 20 years ago — now perhaps you are seeking a bit more structure, underwire cups, wide straps, or a modest tankini. Having said that, I really admire people who have the confidence to let it all hang out, on and off the beach.

Hair Style. Your hair might be a signature style for you, that conveys your personality and individuality. While personal style is important, keep in mind how it might be perceived in a professional capacity. I love the idea of live and let live, just make sure it is acceptable to the setting you will be in.

> **"You can't control the way others see you, but presenting a neat appearance at least doesn't make them pre-judge you before they get to know who you are"**

Different business settings have very different standards of personal appearance and grooming; your haircut if you work in a bank will naturally be quite different from one you might wear if you work at a tattoo parlor! Women and men from various ethnic and cultural backgrounds have different hair types, but whether long and straight, big and curly, straightened or permed or natural or dreads — tame your look a bit for most professional settings. You can always let loose and have fun with your family and friends.

Dressing down. Ripped jeans are for teenagers; on adults, torn clothing looks dirty and messy, like you just didn't have time to pick out something nice to wear. Jeans and denim should be well fitting and in good condition; yoga pants, shorts, t-shirts, and running shoes should be removed immediately after the gym. Freshen up and you will invigorated! When going out to meet friends, it always makes people feel like you value them enough to make an effort to see them. I have found when I am out shopping, even for necessities, or when I am traveling, I get treated better when I am dressed well.

Accessories. An armload of bangles, or long, dangling earrings can look gorgeous, but if they are making noise, it may also be distracting in a business or social setting. If the environment is meant to be quiet, keep it that way. A good start is no more than 3 pieces, so if you have big earrings and a chunky ring, bracelet or watch, then you shouldn't have a brooch or pendant. Choose wisely!

Eyeglasses can also be a fashion accessory with strong vibrant metal or colored plastic frames — or they can disappear into your face, with semi or full rimless versions. Decide which works best for you, and if you have the personality to carry off really strong frames. Or you can change your glasses as you do jewelry, depending on the setting. One of my indulgences is having several pairs of glasses on hand to match my moods and outfits.

Watches can also be a statement piece, a status symbol, or a practical item — although so many people use their cell phones to tell the time now, watches are nearly a thing of the past. Some people use sport watches that count their steps or their pace, and communicate with their phones as well — or just use their phones for that purpose.

Matching shoes, bags, scarves, gloves and hats can be overkill. Tone it down, and accessorize with one great item — you don't want to have red shoes, a red bag, red scarf, and red hat! It's just too much. The saying goes that you can judge an outfit based on the shoes, so keep your shoes in good repair and make sure the look good on you. For men, less is more, and single colors, or monochromatic, makes an outfit look polished, whether dressy or casual. Men and women both should go for beautiful and subtle accessories to complete your look.

Outerwear. Choose coats and jackets for warmth and coverage needed for where you live and what your activities are. Still, there's no need to be a barrel — there are functional and attractive coverups at every length that will let you look good while staying warm. Try various textures, or even a bright color, for something different. If you have a one-time event that requires a coat that you don't need on a regular basis, go to a thrift shop. You will be surprised at what you will find and save money too!

Comfortable, safe, high quality shoes. The highest heels you should wear for your well-being are 2 to 3 inches. That way, you'll actually be able to walk in them, and they'll be comfortable enough to wear all day. If you find with time that your mobility is compromised, there are so many nice styles of slip-on flats that will keep you safe and secure. There's no rule saying you must wear heels; many people wear (or carry) sneakers or flats to work, or to travel to and

My favorite brand of "Good For Your Feet" shoes are SpringStep. They have gorgeous styles for every season and are very well priced, with most styles under $100.00. You can find them at many outlet stores or online at springstep.com. Hush Puppies, Easy Spirit, Clarks, and Vionics also have lines of comfortable, attractive shoes in affordable price ranges.

If your work and social life permit you to wear more casual shoes, visit a running store and get fitted for supportive footwear and insoles that will ensure foot health, reduce bunions, plantar fasciitis and other foot problems. Visit a podiatrist for custom inserts, though these can be pricey; often over-the-counter ones can often solve most issues.

from work. And quality over quantity: buy well-made shoes that will last, rather than cheap knockoffs you will toss after one season.

Outrageous outfits. There is a time and a place for these: Themed events or road races (Super Bowl, Disney), Halloween, a costume party, Carnival in Rio or a Venetian costume ball. That's about it. Otherwise ... leave it for those under 30.

When you do have the appropriate occasion to wear something fun, find an outfit that works for you. Enjoy creating a costume or hunting for one online that shows off your best attributes.

Conclusion

Appearance is not nothing — but it is not everything. Remember that you are more than just what you look like. As time has moved forward, we are getting to a point where women as well as men are being respected for gaining in wisdom and experience with years. A few wrinkles or gray hairs (or even a lot!) are no longer the sign that you are irrelevant or out of touch — rather than you have learned a few things and may have something of value to share.

> **"The wiser mind mourns less for what**
> **age takes away than what it leaves**
> **behind." – William Wordsworth**

Make the best of what you have to offer, both inside and outside. Let your light shine from within, and everyone will like the way you look.

Interactive Chapter Review

Personal Appearance As We Age is Very Personal. What signs of aging have you noticed in yourself? In your friends? In your spouse or significant other? Do any of them particularly bother you? What are they? Have you tried to do anything about them? Has it been effective?

Are there specific physical appearance issues that you think causes other people to judge you for getting older? Has this caused you problems at work? In social settings?

Are there ways in which you have accepted your aging appearance? How does that make you feel?

Do you "go gray" or color your hair? Do you use various hair removal products or services? Why or why not? Would you try a different approach?

Do you dress appropriately for your body type? What style works best for you? Have you considered plastic surgery to change some aspect of your face or body as you age?

Have you felt that your appearance has interfered with your ability to develop relationships with others — work colleagues, friends, lovers? Or have you begun to internalize and find others who know that you cannot judge a book by its cover?

Feeling Good At Any Age. *What are some favorite ways that you maintain a positive frame of mind about aging, despite some of the challenges?*

Do you focus on the ability to move, health and well-being, that implements such as glasses and orthotics are there to help you, what you've learned since you were young, that people who judge you based on your appearance are shallow, not competing with younger people on physical attributes?

What do you do to feel good every day? Dress well? Get a makeover or do regular self-care? What are your favorite ones — massage, facial, haircut, makeup? Or just exercise and good food?

Are you addressing any ongoing or one-time medical issues so you can be at your best? Has doing so allowed you to pursue activities, or inspired those around you to take better care of themselves?

Achieve Your Personal Best. *Do you have inspiring work or hobbies that add joy to your life? Do you feel that helps you to connect with others in a positive way? What do you do to be your personal best? Have you kept up with a lifelong physical activity, or taken up a new one in adulthood?*

Have you spent money to pursue your health and well-being — while avoiding the scams and cons directed against our age group? What have you done? What have you been tempted to do, but thought better and resisted? What have you given in tried, only to learn the hard way was not worth the money?

Do you weigh yourself regularly as a guideline? Are you obsessive and weigh yourself too often, more than once a week? Have you gotten discouraged after a quick weight loss when starting a diet or exercise program and then fallen off track, or do you remain consistent even when at a long plateau?

Fashion for Life. *What is your personal style? Do you find you're still trying to wear clothes you wore 20 years ago, or that people 20 years younger than you are wearing today?*

Have you cleaned out your closet of what no longer works for you or brings you joy? Did you do it alone or ask a friend for help? Have you had a professional bra fitting? Have you gotten rid of your old, dirty, torn, stained clothes? Or taken photos/made a quilt from old t-shirts?

How about color — have you added something to spice up all the black clothes in your closet? What is it? Shirt, shoes, bag, scarf?

Have you had your clothes tailored to fit your shape today? What about style — have you tried something new lately, or are you sticking with what you know works for you?

How about scents, have you tried a new perfume or cologne? Do you remember to apply it lightly, or spray in the air and walk through it? Or do you drench yourself in it?

Are you careful to dress and style your hair appropriately for business settings — and to have fun where appropriate?

Even when you're being more casual, do you keep a bit more covered up than when you were younger? And choose neater clothes — rather than ripped, torn, or workout clothes — for social situations?

How about accessorizing your outfits: do you wear small, simple jewelry, or big statement pieces? Do you wear eyeglasses, and do you have one pair or several for different looks? What about a watch: is it jewelry, a step counter, or do you just use your phone?

Shoes, bags, scarves, hats: do you mix up textures and colors? What colors do you like to use for your accessories? How about for your outerwear? Have you found something functional and flattering? Do you wear heels for certain situations? Or do you prefer flat shoes? What works for you?

Have you had any occasions in the past year to wear some crazy outfit or costume? Do you have a go-to outfit that you wear for Halloween parties? Is it time to look for a new one?

Chapter 8
Managing your Messes:
Are You Oscar or Felix?

Part of living well to age well is having your surroundings in order. This will give you peace of mind. Letting go of the things in your house that you don't need any more is very freeing.

> **"One of the reasons people get old – lose their aliveness – is that they get weighed down by all of their stuff." – Richard Leider**

I cannot emphasis enough how clutter causes confusion as you age, and in many ways prevents you from moving forward. The effect of clutter in your home and office has a profound effect on those around you. There is a fine line between clutter and hoarding. These tendencies increase with age, and can become unhealthy and downright dangerous. Health and safety can be compromised, since many older people may forget where they put important medications or papers, are more likely to trip or fall down in crowded rooms, or knock over valuables stacked on shelves. My siblings and I would always help my parents de-clutter when we went to visit them. It really helped them later on when they couldn't get around as well, and needed the space to function with wheelchairs and walkers.

> **"There are 300,000 items in the average American home." – L.A. Times**

Relationships may suffer as well, as spouses get snappish with each other in cluttered environments for no apparent reason. Friends and family may worry about you, or not want to come visit as often as they would if you had a clean and welcoming home environment, leading to isolation and loneliness, real dangers as we age. Realize that you are also leaving a mess for your heirs to sort through, once you become too infirm or unwell to deal with it yourself, or after you are gone. Even if you have a will, unnecessary stuff causes a terrible strain for the people who have to go through it all and clean it up.

There are many books written on this subject but the method doesn't matter, only you can decide when you are ready to purge. When the time is right for you, plunge in and begin! You may wish to enlist help from family or friends to assist you in decision making. Sometimes it's easier to say goodbye to once-treasured

Keep Your Life Simple

My personal experience is that stuff that causes clutter is paralyzing. Empty out your home so you have room to exercise, eat at a clean table, find what you are looking for easily — and get rid of those diet books, workout videos, and fitness contraptions that you will never use again! In my own home, I live in an "Odd Couple" household, with me being Felix, so I am always negotiating with my husband and daughter to get rid of unnecessary items.

No one I know has a house worthy of Architectural Digest, but even a quick cleanup will make all the difference in how you feel about your surroundings. Having your personal space in order will help you have a calmer and more productive day. One approach is to clean out your house as if you are moving out, and keep only what you absolutely need to get by. You will be astonished at how much extra baggage you have lying around. The worst is when you actually have to move, and you pack up everything but the essentials — and then you don't want to move, because your house is airy and welcoming as opposed to cluttered and oppressive!

possessions that are now cluttering your personal space if you have a chance to say goodbye, tell a story, and share its prior importance with someone else. You can map out your approach and do it room by room (living room, bedroom(s), kitchen, bathroom(s), dining room, pantry, garage, office)... or by item type (clothing, shoes, jackets and coats, books, movies, music, toys and games, electronics, decorative items)... or by area (under the window, bookshelf in the corner, cabinet in the hall, display case, front closet, desk, bureau).

> ## "Keeping baggage from the past will leave no room for happiness in the future..." – Wayne L. Misner

Tips For Items You Want To Let Go

Books that you have read are worth so much more when shared. I love book exchanges or donating them to senior centers or resale stores. Let someone else enjoy a title that meant so much to you. And get rid of those expired travel guides, crumbling paperbacks, school textbooks, and other publications you will never consult again. Keep books on your shelves that you still want to read (or read again), or that spark joy every time you look at the title on the spine.

Magazines that you save for 10 years that have no value should be recycled. If you don't read it within a three-month period it is old news. You can find virtually all of the content online if you decide you want to consult an old recipe or re-read a meaningful article. Send them to the paper recycling bin... or perhaps donate them to a community center, where they can be used for craft work such as collage, decoupage, vision boards, and other cutting-and-pasting projects.

DVDs, VHS tapes, CDs, Cassettes. Do you still have these in your home? It really might be time to let these go. Yes, you invested hundreds — maybe even thousands — of dollars in amassing your collection, but guess what? Do you watch or listen to them anymore? Or are they all just gathering dust on your shelves? Nearly all of us get our media input through streaming services, whether on the TV, car radio, online via our desktop or laptop computers, or on our tablets and cell phones. Alas, even the days when you could sell these for half of their purchase price (or even pennies on the dollar) has passed; perhaps you could donate them to a social service agency that could use them for their clients. (Vinyl record albums are the exception here: there are many websites and collectors that will pay for these — in good condition.)

Toys, Games, Puzzles, Videogames. Do you play them anymore? Is there a regular family game night on your schedule? Do you have children or grandchildren who enjoy them when they visit your house? If not, then those old board games, jigsaw puzzles, crossword puzzles, children's toys — pass them on to the next generation, donate them to a local school, library, or children's center — but get them out of your personal space.

Makeup and Toiletries. I see many of my friends and family members wasting money and space in the bathroom with 5 mascaras, 10 eye pencils, and 15 bottles of shampoos in the shower. You may have a stack of electric shavers (most that don't work), rusty razors, old shower heads, and shelves full of soaps and expired creams and lotions. I have a tendency to hoard those single use sample and travel size items you get at hotels. Get rid of all it and only keep what you need for personal grooming. The biggest secret about personal care items is that if you have less, you use it more often and more regularly.

The other reason you may have so many beauty products is because they are your connection to your youth. You should know your own personal "look" by now, so chances are you don't use most of what you have. Anti-aging creams don't really work in the long term. Trust me, I have tried them all, so don't waste your money... and toss those ones you've been using sparingly, they're probably long expired.

Kitchen/Pantry. Throw out those 10 year old bottles of herbs and spices. They have lost their potency and might even have bugs in them. Get rid of the diet products and canned goods that have expired. Many of us come from times when food or money was tight, or it was hard to get to the store, and we keep our homes stocked with enough food to hold us for a month or more. Be sure to cycle your oldest food to the front of the cabinet, and re-stock from the back, so you don't end up with expired cans hiding in the corner. The only exception to this is keeping a well-stocked emergency preparedness kit somewhere other than the kitchen, but make sure you keep that current as well.

And no, you won't become the gourmet cook you always dreamed of being by having tons of kitchen equipment. Clean and organize the items that you use, and give away the rest. Stop buying kitchen gadgets and fancy specialty cookware for yourself that you think you might need later — you will probably only use them once, if at all!

Cleaning Products. And speaking of cleaning — how many cleaning products do you really need? It might be time to clean out the ancient copper cleaner under your sink, and neaten up that area as well. Most of us have far more soap, bleach, ammonia, vinegar, glass cleaner, sink cleaner, steel wool, sponges, towels, etc. than we could ever use. Again, organize it, know what you have so you don't buy duplicates, and keep them safe from visiting children or grandchildren. Offer your surplus to a neighbor that might be in need.

Dishes/Glasses. One great tip for your dining area as you age is using plastic tableware — not the disposable kind that you buy in a party store, but good, reusable, durable plastic dishes. Melamine

---

Eat well tip
Many of us still hold onto the belief that a full refrigerator and a well-stocked pantry is a sign of wealth. As we get older, that can very quickly turn into hoarding, and food going bad. If having empty shelf space where you usually keep food bothers you, consolidate your dry goods into one kitchen cabinet and use the others for non-food items such as linens, paper goods, and office supplies. It's a great use of space and keeps the overall clutter at a minimum.

---

looks almost as good as fine china and is very safe. It washes well and is relatively inexpensive. You can find some fabulous patterns with lots of inventory at Target and Dollar Stores nationwide. Silicone wine glasses and thermal cups are fantastic and reusable, and eliminate the dangers of broken glass. Unfortunately, spills and falls are more common as we age due to diminished balance and grip strength, and it is better to start preparing now for your later years. I outfitted my parents' house with beautiful reusable plastic dishware, and it helped to keep them safe.

Papers. I understand the need we all seem to have to keep every school essay, every book report, every set of grades that the kids earned. If the kids aren't interested in the originals, you can photograph them and scan them to save in an album. How about old stationery and post cards, tax returns and receipts? You only need to save the past 7 years or receipts and records in case of a tax audit. Before that, you can keep the return itself (or again, scan and save it electronically), and receipts for big-ticket items (appliances, furniture, automobiles, boats, artwork, jewelry) — but other than that, get rid of all that paper!

Electronics. Do you have an old phone, cell phone, digital camera (or film camera!), cassette players, CD players, MP3 players, etc., in the top of your closet? Dozens of remotes for TVs and stereos that are long gone? And speaking of papers — how about the instructions and warranty cards for all of those old TVs, VCRs, DVD players and other electronic gadgets? Or for those kitchen appliances you never use anymore? Vanished blenders, mixers, waffle makers, toaster ovens, microwaves? Time to say farewell to all of this clutter at last.

Furniture. Have you been holding on to extra pieces to help your children when they set up their own homes? An old couch, dining table, curtains and drapes, carpets? Perhaps it's time to let these go. The days when furniture, like clothing, was an expensive investment are long past, and many young people don't even like the styles of furniture that we have been saving for them for so long. Check to be sure they don't want them, and then say farewell — perhaps pass them along to a local shelter that could make good use of them.

Holiday Decorations. I have a friend who stores her extensive collection of holiday décor in a rented storage area in the basement of her co-op, for which she pays $50 per month. That adds up to $600 per year, much more than she would pay to purchase brand new decorations every year! Of course, there are some heirloom items she doesn't want to get rid of, but they are a small portion of what is stored there. Even if you don't have a similar financial savings by getting rid of your décor, you can trim back what you keep so that it doesn't clutter up your day-to-day living space, or the top and back of your closet areas.

> **"One out of every 10 Americans rent offsite storage, the fastest growing segment of the commercial real estate industry over the past four decades." – New York Times Magazine**

Clothes. Get rid of clothes that don't fit, clothes that are stained or torn, clothes you never wear, and definitely get rid of clothes with tags on them. Are you hoping some classic piece may come back into fashion? Good luck with that; even "vintage" styles get re-done when they come back on the runway, the original version just looks dowdy. Has your style changed, but you keep your old clothes around anyway because they remind you of the way you used to like dressing? Time to let them go and move on. Do you keep a safe pair of "fat pants" around in case you put on a few pounds? You may wish to reconsider that approach...

Housewares. Sheets, towels, curtains, bedding, drapes — they should be clean, neat, in good repair, and in regular rotation, or they have no business being in your house. As noted elsewhere, many of us come from a time when these items were expensive and precious, and therefore we are loathe to let them go.

Perhaps you have a blanket that was knitted by your mother or grandmother, or some handmade lace or crocheted table covers — you might wish to preserve a few of these for your children, but if they are not interested, it might be time to

Swedish Death Cleaning
As horrible as it sounds, this is actually a very positive mindset. In The Gentle Art of Swedish Death Cleaning: How to free yourself and your family of a lifetime of clutter, author Margareta Magnusson encourages the reader to embrace the process of clearing out belongings so that others won't have to do it after you are gone.

The Swedish word "dostadning" means to slowly de-clutter as you age, preferably starting when you are young enough to handle it, and keeping throughout the years. Magnusson also suggests sharing the process with your friends and family so everyone understands what you are doing, and what you want done with what is left. Keep in mind that what you hold dear might be meaningless to your heirs — but hearing a story from you might fill the objects with memory. Lastly, after purging, try to reward yourself with self-care and relaxing activities instead of going shopping!

pass these along. Is there a historical society or local shop that would be interested in such handmade crafts? That would let them give pleasure and use to someone, rather than be vulnerable to dust and moths in storage.

> "It is best as one grows older to strip oneself of possessions, to shed oneself downward like a tree, to be almost wholly earth before one dies." – Sylvia Townsend Warner

How to talk to yourself about the purging process

Are you clinging to stuff that you might come in handy someday? Does it have sentimental value even though you no longer use it? Remember: if something you have in your home were necessary, you would be using it. If not, get rid of it. Sometimes looking back on old items is not nostalgic, it is melancholy. You may wish to be free of certain memories.

"Hanging on to things we no longer need is like extra weight, it keeps us stuck and unable to move freely through life"

Keep in mind you are also burdening your heirs with too much inventory for them to clean up when you are no longer here. If it's something you think they would enjoy, give it to them now! There's no time like the present, and you will still be here to enjoy their gratitude for receiving a thoughtful gift.

"Average Americans spend one year of their life looking for lost or misplaced items." – U.S. News and World Report

Often when we have clutter and own too much stuff, we cannot find what we need and end up buying another one, so now you have two of the same unused items, which is really a waste of money. Keep what you need, organize it and label it so you can locate it when needed — and get rid of the rest.

Start out by getting rid of duplicates of things you have, or items which no longer work. Several sets of dishes, two copies of the same book, a closet full of unmatched (or broken) luggage, purses or jackets with bad zippers, drawers filled with pens, pencils, tape, string, staples, etc.

Garages and attics across the world are filled with unused and unseen items. I know that your individual collection represents a lifetime and maybe many generations, but the items are useless if they are not being enjoyed. If items have been in storage for over a year, get rid of them whether you sell them, give them as gifts, donate them to a charity, recycle them, or throw them in the garbage: they are not serving your life today.

"Twenty-five percent of people with two-car garages don't have room to park cars inside them and 32% only have room for one vehicle." – U.S. Department of Energy

Getting rid of items you know longer use or need will help you appreciate what you do keep, and will keep you in the present. Honoring and remembering your parents and grandparents can be done with just a few items and photos.

Another thing I like to do when I'm ready to get rid of something like childhood artwork or a favorite stuffed animal: take a digital photo of it, maybe even with the artist, now all grown up! Then you'll have the memory forever, without having it clutter up space in your closet or in your guest bedroom.

Start small, as noted above, one room at a time, one category at a time, one area at a time. Or you could try the fun "23-skidoo!" method: walk around your house with an empty laundry basket and choose 23 items that you can get rid of right now! Used candles, old electrical extension cords, chipped coffee mugs, dog-eared paperbacks, torn underwear — pick any 23 items from any room, any category, any area, and get them out of your house immediately. You'll be amazed how easy it is to come up with 23 items you truly do not need and will not miss. It is freedom.

What To Do With The Stuff You're Letting Go

For items of value, you can offer them to friends, family, shelters, organizations such as the Salvation Army or Goodwill — anywhere that someone else can use them is a good way to go. You can do an internet search for "places to donate things" and get a dozen results in just a few seconds!

There are often hospices, halfway houses, homeless shelters, and other social service agencies in your community that would be grateful for donations of lightly used sheets and towels, books and magazines, even decorative items for the common areas, staff offices, or residents' rooms.

If you are up to the task (or are willing to ask for some help in the process), you can list the items on resale websites and maybe make some money back. Another possibility is to get booth space at a flea market to re-coup some money, or give your old kitchen wares or home furnishings to a young family just starting out.

Perhaps your own children, grandchildren, nieces or nephews could make active use of your unwanted furniture, tools, kitchen or garden items as they set up their household. If you don't have your own family of the next generation, check with a local YMCA or other family organization to see if their members could use some of these items. Donated cribs, baby carriages, bikes, and children's furniture are always welcome to new families.

As noted above, items of value could be given as gifts. Do you have jewelry you no longer wear, too many prints or paintings to display in your home? Giving these as holiday or birthday presents is a lovely way to share something you care about with those close to you, and save on the expense of buying presents as well. Make the gift extra-special by writing up or telling the story of the item's history.

Positive and Negative Psychological Effects of Purging

Beware that there may be a withdrawal period from when you rid yourself of stuff, and possibly even a craving to have these items back — or to replace them with more junk. If you can fight the urge to restock your house with things you don't need, these feelings will pass and you will find a new sense of freedom in traveling lightly.

Do you feel joy or sorrow when you look at your belongings? The items that don't make you feel happy should go. Author Marie Kondo, the author of *The Life-Changing Magic Of Tidying Up*, and host of the related series on Netflix, made a lifelong study of organization and came up with some brilliant solutions:

Keep ONLY stuff that sparks joy

We think we should rely on our rational mind instead of intuition. The opposite is true. Sparking joy cannot be explained

Don't focus on what to discard... focus on what to keep

A gift is not a "thing;" rather it is a means to convey emotions. Once it's done this job, it can be discarded if you don't love it

Letting go is much more important than getting

Just like overeating, overspending is trying to stave off stress. But both cause more stress

A home free of clutter is a home filled with light

The Kondo method addresses five areas: clothing, books, paper, "miscellaneous" (which covers kitchen/bathroom/garage) and finally sentimental items. One of the unique facets of her approach to letting go is first, thanking your home for providing shelter and protection (which leads you to feeling it is worthwhile to tend to it and keep it tidy), and second, thanking the items that you let go, for providing service or value while you owned them. This

Eat well tip
While cleaning out your home, be sure to take care of yorself, eat something energizing and hydrate well. This can be physically exhausting and emotionally taxing work. It is important to treat yourself gently and nurture yourself while you are freeing yourself from the burdens of what you have acquired over the decades. Take time during the process to sit down, have a relaxing cup of tea or a glass of iced water with lemon, and enjoy the process — and the results!

gentle system allows one to move on with a minimum of painful attachment and loss.

If this all is very hard for you, ask a friend or family member to come and help you go through and separate from your possessions. An outside eye will not have the emotional attachment that you have to these things, and may help you see what is getting in the way of your discarding them. Sometimes just telling someone about why you are attached to something, and why it was important to you, gives you the freedom to let it go at last.

Many people have also had success with the gentle and supportive baby steps of the **FlyLady** approach, by Maria Cilley, author of **Sink Reflections**. Her website and app provide many tips to address CHAOS (Can't Have Anyone Over Syndrome), including:

Shine your sink

Lay out clothes for tomorrow

Get dressed to lace-up shoes

Declutter for 15 minutes a day

Preventing New Accumulation

Sometimes there is a tendency, when we clean out our homes, to go out and buy new things — the need to be surrounded by items is that strong! Going forward, before you buy anything new, ask yourself: Does this spark joy? Do I really need this? Is it practical? Will it cause clutter? Can I afford it? Why am I buying this?

Or use the replacement program: if you buy a new pair of shoes, get rid of an old pair to make room for them. Ditto for clothes, kitchen gadgets, electronics — if you buy something new, you must get rid of something old in the same category, to assure that you do not end up with fresh clutter.

Another approach is to step away from a potential purchase for 24 hours and think about it. Chances are you don't need it, it might duplicate something you already have, and it may be a waste of money. At a certain point, don't buy anything new unless you absolutely need it! Investing in your future should be in the form of saving, not spending, seeking out new experiences, not things.

Those items that once defined us become little more than dust collectors as we age.

"Americans spend $1.2 trillion annually on nonessential goods — in other words, items they do not need." – The Wall Street Journal

As noted above, one fabulous way to take advantage of new technology is to take digital photographs of things that you once loved and served you, that you want to now let go of and bring joy to someone else. You can store these photos on CDs, flash drives, or in the cloud, so they literally take up zero space in your home. This allows you to go back and look at the photos of these items, so you can reminisce with happy memories of times gone by, without feeling bogged down by the physical items cluttering up your personal space today.

Interactive Chapter Review

Clearing the Clutter. Is your house in order? Are you surrounded by clutter? Do you have underlying organization, or do you sweep messes "under the rug?

Do you suffer from psychological or emotional concerns due to the condition of your home? Does it affect your relationships? Are you concerned about your safety in navigating your residence, as far as falls or knocking things over?

Have you consulted any books or TV shows about how to conquer clutter? Have you begun to implement any new methods to improve your situation? If not, are you ready to take the plunge?

Do you like to approach clearing clutter by room, by item type, or by area? Or do you do it haphazardly, here and there as it strikes you — or all at once, in an all-out attack? Which is the easiest area for you do deal with — the bedroom? Bathroom? Kitchen? Garage? Which is the hardest and why?

Tips for What to Let Go. *What is hardest for you to sort through and let go? Books? Magazines? Movies and Music? Toys and games? Makeup and Toiletries? Cooking supplies and gadgets? Tableware? Papers? Electronics? Furniture and décor? Holiday decorations? Clothing? Housewares? Mementos and other sentimental items?*

What has gotten in the way of your clearing your clutter? Do you justify it by saying it may be useful in the future? Or you don't want to lose precious memories of the past? Does it help to think that you are making it easier for others who will not have to clean up after you later, when you are unable to deal with it yourself, or gone? Could you make gifts of items you are holding onto for your children today?

Have you ever bought a second copy of something that you already own because you couldn't find it? Can you easily get rid of duplicate or broken items right away? Can you take photographs of special things and say farewell to them?

What groups or organizations could make use of the items you no longer need? Who could these things serve and bring joy to today? Can you sell them online or at a local secondhand or resale shop? What about giving special items as gifts, along with their story?

Psychological Effects of Purging. *Are you afraid you will miss the things you give away, and possibly rush out to buy new stuff to take its place? Can you try the replacement system to prevent new accumulation?*

Have you tried saying "thank you" to your home for taking care of you, and to the items which you are giving away, to make the transition easier? Have you asked for help from a friend or family member in getting through this process of letting go?

Chapter 9
Relationships As We Age

As we age, surrounding ourselves with people who make us feel good about ourselves helps us to feel safe and secure.

The value in having a lifelong (or long-term) partner, a few meaningful long-standing friendships, and cordial relations with all those we meet, far outweighs any short-term gratification of playing the field or having superficial contacts with a large number of people. Everyone I have ever interviewed about what they valued most, always talk about quality, lifelong companionship, and deep connections, with a spouse, family, and close friends.

Are you married? Single? Divorced? Widowed? Once you check the box that applies to you, think about how your marital status makes you feel. Proud, empowered, embarrassed, sad? Relationships have many faces and there are all kinds of arrangements out there. Do what works for you. If you are in search of a mate, and are having trouble finding someone that strikes your fancy, go back to the drawing board and evaluate your approach. Are you looking for what you need or want, both, neither?

Your family, friends, pets, work environment, and level of physical contact with the outside world all play a role in how you interact with people. The more you put yourself out there, the higher the risk, but the rewards are many and having loved ones around for the rest of your life is priceless. Even if you find that you are having to re-establish relationships late in life or starting over again, it will be highly beneficial for you and your extended family. Think of the celebration of happiness and unity in the Sister Sledge song title, "*We Are Family.*"

The Benefits of Family

A person's family should be the one safe haven that he or she can always rely on. If all else fails, it is very comforting to know we will always be welcomed by parents, adult children, and relatives who are part of our extended family. When we reach that point where our parents are infirm or gone, we all want to recreate that sense of security that a family brings. In the absence of this we can feel very insecure, isolated, and alone.

"When you get to my age, you'll really measure your success in life by how many of the people you want to have love you actually do love you." – Warren Buffett

For those of us who have significant losses or estrangement from our immediate family, creating a "family of choice" can provide a loving alternative. Often used by gay people in past generations, when ostracized by blood relations, everyone can learn from this pattern and build a family with intention among people of like interests. Note that a "family of choice" is different than a circle of friends — friendships may come to an end, and people grow apart, whereas a family of choice will stick together even when there are differences and disagreements.

"You are the average of the 5 people you spend the most time with." – Jim Rohn

Look back in Chapter 1 at the section on the Blue Zones: Okinawans in Japan chose a group of 5 people early on, and forge bonds with them that lasts a lifetime. This can be done at any age, and can often support lifestyle choices and changes. You may create a family-like bond with friends from your yoga class, a nutritional program like Weight Watchers, your local running group or sports team, or a recovery group such as A.A., and have resources to turn to when you are feeling challenged. This can also affect your own success in life, as motivational speaker Jim Rohn has noted that, "You are the average of the 5 people you spend the most time with."

Family Issues

We all have family members that we love and hate. In some cases we feel both of those emotions at once. Growing up without a healthy family dynamic results in self-esteem issues for many people, and as I said earlier, we make most of our decisions based on our emotional health at that time and place. If a family member is truly unbearable, you may wish to reduce contact to a minimum and seek out loved ones who you can rely on. (Now you can see the value of creating that "family of choice"!) It is important not to subject yourself to constant negative judgment, belittling, criticism, prejudice, hostility, nagging, fighting, or other aspects of a toxic relationship. Over time, this can erode your own sense of self, and may even result in your treating others the same way. Use your own good judgment for when you may have to gently remove yourself, and love these difficult family members from afar.

However, if possible, staying in touch with our families — even if the relationships are not ideal — will give you a sense of security, in case you ever need to rely on them later on in life. Remember that we all change and grow during the course of our lives, and difficult relationships with parents or siblings or cousins when we were younger may change and evolve as we develop and mellow with age. It might be worth re-contacting family members with whom you had conflict years ago — you are no longer the same person, and neither are they!

"Social relationships have as much impact on physical health as blood pressure, smoking, physical activity, and obesity." – American Society on Aging

It is time-consuming and challenging to maintain good relationships with family members, both those with whom we enjoy spending time, and those with whom we have a bad history. Be careful not to let the shadow of "obligation" or "duty" fall over your attempts to reach out; let a sense of joy and exploration color your initiatives and responses to invitations for family events. This leads to success more often than stiff, wooden communications which imply you are only doing this because you should, not because you want to. If you are someone who finds it easy to be kind to strangers, but harder to care for those closest to you, remember: charity begins at home.

Often we don't reveal the truth about our lives to family members for fear that they will perceive us as a burden — or worse yet, that we will expose the fact that we are not perfect. If you are able to repair broken relationships with family members, I say give it a try. It's a better alternative than living with the strain of not knowing where you stand, not having a support system, and possibly regretting your estrangement after they are gone and there's no chance to rebuild anymore.

The Importance of Friendships

We all have a variety of friends that come from the different stages in our lives. We have the childhood friend that we will never give up, even if we outgrow the relationship. The work friend with whom we commiserate or celebrate with about what's going on at our jobs. The fellow parents at your child's school. Gym or yoga or craft or travel buddies with whom we share common interests and activities. Each relationship is unique, and often your friends are not friends with each other. The only time they get to meet is when you have a big get-together and invite your separate groups of friends.

It is very rare that a group of friends stay close forever. That is a myth that movies and TV shows perpetuate. Often friendships dissolve over time due to lack of communication, changing interests, geographic distance — and yet we always hold a special place in our hearts for our old friends. When the friendship is no longer working, or we lose touch, we feel so sad. Nothing is worse than having a friend turn on you after years of friendship... though if you are honest with yourself, you may see that the friendship was never that great and the blow up was usually a long time coming.

"True friendships don't end because of time and distance apart"

Look at your life now: do you have a handful of good, close friends? This is very important. Keep in mind that going forward your friends will become your lifeline. Only let in the people that you can rely on, and who make you feel good about yourself. (As noted above, that includes your family members whose behavior and treatment of you may not serve your best interests.) Just like cultivating relationships with family, keeping up friendships takes time and attention — and you don't want to be spending that investment in a place where you will not get a good (emotional) return for your efforts.

I spend a lot of time socializing because it makes me feel whole. I have friends throughout the world who I stay in touch with via social media, and whenever we happen to be in the same city we get together and catch up. I spend time with childhood friends because we have a bond that is strong as super glue and I know we can always rely on each other. I have made friends in recent years that have blossomed into very close relationships — and I have lost some people along the way who I thought were friends but they had other ideas. I'm also incredibly fortunate that I am very close with all of my siblings, and we are in touch on a regular basis as well. I don't always get what I need out of every friendship, but I believe that everyone has something to offer and each person is worth a try. I am always inspired when I think of the Carole King song title, "You've Got a Friend."

If you feel that you want — or need! — to get out and meet more people, try organizing a reunion or a friendly get-together that has a theme. Card games, book clubs, sports leagues, fitness centers, and religious or spiritual groups are all wonderful ways to meet people with shared interests. I just joined a book club and found a great group of like-minded ladies to hang out with once a month.

Much to my surprise, many people have found that new connections with people can be built online, through social media and shared interest groups. It is so easy to reach out and reconnect with old friends you haven't seen in years, and you may find out that the friendship can start up as though no time has passed. New acquaintances that start out online often develop in real life — I have made many new connections through my online running groups that have blossomed into real friendships.

Romance and Dating in the New Century

If you are single, and want to find companionship, you need to set your own rules. We've all heard those lines passed down from generation to generation about how to get a spouse and keep him or her. I bet you think those rules have served you pretty well up until now. Well, forget everything you thought you knew about dating. The times have changed, and that means we have to change, too.

"In order to trust someone else, you have to trust yourself"

The rules are what you make them. Dating should be a shared experience with both parties fully participating. Before you go out and get too involved, have an honest discussion about what you are both looking for. It is important to compromise, but don't give up who you are or jeopardize your life just to have companionship, you are worth much more than that. Be cautious that at this stage you are not being viewed as a "nurse or a purse," but regarded as a full human being.

Both parties can be equally responsible for the cost of dates and what activities you would like to do. You don't need to play games with phone numbers and who calls first or how long it takes to call back or return a text or email. If there is mutual interest it will work itself out. Getting back to being yourself at all times will help you find someone that is truly suited for you, rather than continuing to set up yourself and the people you are dating for disappointment.

Going out on a date? Or even just out to lunch with a friend, or a group? Business meeting, job interview, potential client? Are you

Eat well tip
When dining out with a new friend or business associate that you would like to impress, be careful not to compromise everything you have worked for physically and emotionally to seal the deal. It's okay to eat within the parameters of what works for you, regardless of the pressure to drink and indulge. It is always best to be the one who is clear and sober at the end of the day.

the client? Clarify ahead of time who is paying or how you will split the bill, and speak your mind if you are uncomfortable about the location, price, time, and or date. Everything is negotiable. If the other party is inflexible, that will tell you a lot as well, and you should pay attention. Let intuition be your guide: go by your gut feel, it will always be right.

We were all told no sex on the first date. This is a good rule so you can get to know each other without feeling bad if it doesn't work out, and reduce your risk of any health repercussions. If after a number of dates the relationship seems to be going well, then you decide when is the right time. If you aren't knocked out when you first kiss, give it time, that spark isn't always there in the beginning, sometimes attraction grows with the relationship.

As noted above: if your gut tells you he or she is not the one, follow it. Real love with commitment and genuine friendship doesn't play out like a romantic movie. When its working, have all the sex you want, when you can, at any age. It is good, healthy, and fun, and keeps you young.

Those of us who remember when dating was often a chance meeting or an introduction through friends, family and work, tend to feel that online dating is for losers who have no social life. It is now regarded as a great way to meet people with shared interests, but without too much up-front commitment. Try it (with common-sense caution) — you never know who you will meet!

And as always, don't try to be someone you're not in order to attract a romantic partner. Some people will like you no matter what, and some will dislike you no matter what — you might as well have the ones who like you actually like the "real" you, rather than some phony self you try to project to impress other people. That's not to say you shouldn't present your best self, you don't want to be a slob or speak poorly or hastily — but hopefully you don't even do that on your own, you want to respect and enjoy your own company yourself.

If you are going to live with someone — whether platonically, romantically, or legally — establish a plan for your finances, what expenses you are splitting, what you keep separate, etc. A written contract is best, if for no other reason than you can go back and look at what you agreed upon in case the situation goes sour. It is always in your best interest to protect yourself.

If and when you do enter a new relationship, remember that both parties may have become more "set in their ways" over the years. Don't expect to be in perfect harmony in your living arrangements, lifestyle, habits, likes and dislikes. While you should always treat each other with consideration and respect (indeed, of either of these are lacking, get out!) — but give each other space to be yourselves, and do things the way each of you like to do them. Many people who start new relationships later in life continue to maintain separate residences, finances, vacations, and groups of friends. While it may be true that "two can live as cheaply as one," that savings may not be worth it if sharing space causes friction or disharmony in an otherwise positive relationship.

"Grow old along with me! The best is yet to be." – Robert Browning

Long (Long) Term Romantic Relationships

Not much is written about the challenges — and delights — of very long term romantic relationships. Perhaps you met your spouse in college — or were high school sweethearts — maybe you even met as children. How do you keep romance alive after 20, 30, 40, 50 years with the same person? How do you prevent the "seven-year itch" or a mid-life crisis from destroying a beautiful relationship?

Relationships are complicated, and unfortunately so many long term marriages end very late in the game. This is due to a breaking point after many years of unhappiness and strife. Many couples do stay together until death due to habit, fear of being alone, religious beliefs, or financial concerns.

Although these circumstances, good and bad, may all play a role in a lifelong partnership, I truly believe the secret to a happy long term life together is communicating who you really are to your partner. It is even more basic than what you want and what you need. Raw honesty in everything you do forges the bonds of a great relationship, especially if you are true to yourself. Remember the story of the Piña Colada Song? They never knew they had common interests because neither one ever bothered to ask!!

As an example, in terms of being a morning person vs. a night person, or a social butterfly vs. a hermit, my husband and I are complete opposites. I am up late at night and sleep late in the morning, while my husband is buzzing about at the crack of dawn. I am very social, while he can generously be described as a hermit. Early on, these differences caused conflict, but we made incredible strides in our relationship because we discussed these differences, were honest with each other (and ourselves) about our preferences, and we figured out how and when to do things separately and together.

"Those who love deeply never grow old; they may die of old age, but they die young." - Ben Franklin

When a long term relationship goes sour, how often do we see the War of the Roses, with no-holds-barred attacks on each other? This kind of negativity ages us, makes us pinched and hostile and distrustful, not attractive to anyone, or even ourselves. How do we prevent reaching that point of no return, where revenge and hatred dictate all of the decisions made? Even if you do drift apart, there are ways of maintaining the relationship while redefining the terms. You can stay married and share a household but sleep in separate rooms and carry on essentially separate lives. You can also make financial arrangements that are designed to benefit both of you without strings attached, rather than each party trying to punish the other.

Many divorces are blamed on the proverbial mid-life crisis for both men and women. The mid-life crisis often comes at a time, on an average at 45 years old, when we can still envision changing the course of our lives. Many of us ponder our lives at a certain point, and it's not necessarily a crisis, but a re-evaluation of where we are at in life. At a much older age, there are less options for starting anew. At any point in the relationship couples can go through this re-evaluation process together, by communicating their fears, disappointments and hopes for the future as a unit. Couples counseling can be very valuable at this stage, if both parties are committed to finding the best way to move into the future. Hopefully working together in this way will lead to more bonding going forward rather than estrangement.

"Maintaining honest, open relationships keeps us feeling young"

The benefits of a long-term romantic relationship are numerous. Working through your differences and getting to a point of mutual trust leads to unconditional love and complete security. Ups and downs are normal, and sticking it out has to do with tolerance for the differences, compromising, and embracing the good aspects.

Living Space/Arrangements As We Age

One measure of success in our society is having a larger house, preferably with lots of land. This is a crowning achievement, but can be very isolating socially. As we get into our 4th, 5th, and 6th decades, our losses of loved ones through death, divorce, and moving become more prevalent. As much as you love your house and the memories are priceless, if you find yourself empty-nesting or living alone in a big house, think about moving to a more populated area, preferably where you know people or can meet them more easily and create a strong local support community. As the Beatles song title reminds us, we can get by "With a little help from my friends."

Even for couples, changing your residence as you age is common. Planning for the future when you may be less agile than you are now, perhaps you want to look for a single-level home so you don't have the challenge of running up and down stairs every day. You might wish to move into a planned community or a condo so you don't have the heavy chores and expenses of roof repair, lawn care, and so on. These often have community centers, too, where you can meet and enjoy activities with other people from your generation. We have all heard that not being completely alone, having a pet, and living with other people is healthier and safer. It is also reassuring to know you can knock on a neighbor's door if you need anything. You can have a walking or movie buddy, or at the very least just someone to talk to.

Many older people shun the idea of roommates, but this can actually be a great set-up. You save money and have constant, built-in companionship. Two adults decide to live together to share expenses and to have someone around to rely on. I love this concept, and it can be adapted for all ages. Having a roommate is widely viewed as something you grow out of, so drop your preconceived notions and start sharing!

A small word of caution: **"I can see clearly now"** should be your mantra! Make sure when you embark on a new relationship, especially a live-in one, that you get clarification about everything. Don't assume anything going in. You might go back to some tried-and-true methods of sharing space that you

Is Shared Housing Right For You?

Remember the Golden Girls? According to Seniorly. com, a 2012 Census Bureau survey showed that over a third of women in the US who are 65 or older live alone. One of the reasons cited in the survey is that the divorce rate for people over 50 has doubled since 1990, and other reasons include the death of a spouse or the choice to remain independent.

As the challenges and costs of independent living become more difficult, the roommate option can be increasingly attractive, enabling people to stay in their homes and find interesting companions in the process.

Various sources online and through other forms of media report that senior roommate situations can be far better than living alone.

did when you were younger, like a chore chart to ensure that everything is handled in a fair manner, so that you (or your roommates) don't get stuck always cleaning the kitchen, or the bathroom, or taking out the trash.

Going It Alone

If you want to stay in your home — by yourself, no roommates or family — and not move to an apartment or senior community, put together a plan to help yourself.

> If you are up to the task, get a dog or cat, they are amazing and will keep you company. Remember that dogs need walking in all weathers, and will have to be boarded if you travel, which can be expensive. Cats need care when you're out of town as well, and both require veterinary care and daily interaction.

> Ask a neighbor to help you with household repairs, and see if there are local teens that will come and help with chores in exchange for community service credit. This is a win/win for everyone. If this is not available, find a number for a local "handy person" who will be will be on call — as well as skilled tradespeople like plumbers and electricians and locksmiths as needed.

> Make sure you have a regular schedule of when you will check in with family or friends so they know you are all right. This is a good plan even for young people who live on their own. In my 20s I had a best friend who got very mad at me if I didn't check in with her (or check on her) every day!

> Don't be embarrassed to have a life alert button. They are available as a necklace, wristband or can be attached to a belt. I have family members who were stranded for hours without help because they would not or could not call anyone, especially not the EMTs.

If you run or bike outdoors, wear an ID tag like Road ID, and a medic alert bracelet if needed. That way, in case or an emergency, people know how to contact your family, and are aware of any medical conditions you may have.

Keep a current list of all emergency contacts visible in the house; a list of your health care providers and medications, if any; and keep a file of all of your advance directives nearby.

If at some point you decide that you are ready to move into any form of a care facility, start the conversation with a social worker at your local hospital, religious institution, or call Medicare directly and get help in making these decisions. Some assisted living homes provide the option for you to pay full cost for a set number of years, and then be assured of lifetime care. They provide tiered levels of assistance from minimal, to help with daily living, to medical and hospice care. Prepare for these expenses well in advance, or talk with your adult children and other family members to see if they can help. Sometimes financial contributions are easier for them than having to provide personal care and attention as we begin to need more assistance. (See below for more information about end of life care.)

"He who is of a calm and happy nature will hardly feel the pressure of age, but to him who is of an opposite disposition, youth and age are equally a burden." - Plato

Psychological Growth

Take a good hard look at your personality type — are you hyperactive, defensive, and driven? These behaviors (that might have worked in your favor when you were in your thirties) will turn on you as you age. I am not suggesting you slow down, but aggressive behavior doesn't work well when you are forging relationships later in life. Yes, it is very hard for classic "Type A" personalities to dial down and temper, but it is very important as

Loneliness Can Be Dangerous

Be aware! While many who may prefer to live alone feel that they prefer having control over their living space, or are genuine introverts who recharge best in their own company — research has shown that loneliness can contribute to decline and death:

"Researchers at the University of California, San Francisco found that loneliness plays a large role in the decline so often associated with old age. The study followed 1,600 adults, with an average age of 71 — despite controlling for socioeconomic status and health, the lonely consistently held higher mortality rates. Nearly 23% of lonely participants died within six years of the study, as opposed to only 14% of those that reported adequate companionship."

"Another study, from the Public Library of Science, reported that elderly people who don't have enough social interaction are twice as likely to die prematurely. To put it in perspective, the increased mortality risk is comparable to the death risk of smoking. Loneliness is approximately twice as dangerous as obesity." (Cited from www.healthyfoodhouse.com, 1/16/2019)

you age to be fully engaged in personal relationships. Develop an adaptive coping style, and always try to stay optimistic. Take it easy, give people the benefit of the doubt, "don't sweat the small stuff," as the saying goes. A negative outlook is reflected on our facial expression even more as we grow older, and can be a fast turn-off to new friendships; people don't want to be around an angry, hostile, critical, resentful sourpuss. You don't want to go through life alone.

If you tend to be passive and a people-pleaser, you have the opposite problem. Friends, family, and work colleagues walk all over you, acquaintances (and con men) take advantage of your soft heart and easygoing nature — and this only gets worse as you age, when people with ill intentions really target you as an easy mark. Do not be polite if you are being wronged! You cannot get this time back and you need to fight the battles when you can. If you hold your tongue when you know you someone is trying to put one over on you, what may happen is that you will lash out somewhere else — and harm a good relationship instead. Now is the time to begin to stand up for yourself. Ask for help from close family or friends if you are worried that someone may be trying to take advantage of you, financially or emotionally.

When you understand how your behavior affects others, and don't hurt anyone else in the process, you truly are free to be yourself. And if you see things about yourself that you realize are affecting others in a negative way, perhaps you would like to change them. Never say an old dog can't learn new tricks; if you are motivated and put your mind to it, you can achieve things you never imagined at any age. Try having a smile on your face even at rest. Try saying something nice to a stranger at a mall or a restaurant, or to a longtime friend or family member. You'd be amazed at what a kind word can do.

"Changing the way you think is hard, and changing the way you act is even harder"

That's not to say that it's easy. Pushing the limits in every aspect of our lives seems natural except when it comes to our psychological growth. Most people don't address what is wrong in life until a crisis happens, and even then the denial can be so overwhelming, we don't do anything about it. Read some inspiring books, join a self-help group, consider counseling or spiritual explorations — begin to work on yourself in ways that your busy life never allowed you to do in the past. This is your time for personal growth and development, revel in it.

Listen to your instincts and intuition, but "check your work" with a trusted friend or advisor. When a current situation doesn't work for you, whether it is personal or professional, see it as a challenge and try a new approach. "If you always do what you've always done, you will always get what you've always gotten." Look deep inside yourself for answers, they are all there. Learn to trust yourself. If you'd like some outside support to help you get in touch with that inner wisdom, consider seeking out a professional mentor or hiring a business coach, or working with an experienced counselor or life coach to address personal changes you'd like to make. Many successful people have coaches in their lives.

"The older I grow, the more I distrust the familiar doctrine that age brings wisdom." – H. L. Mencken

When the midlife crisis hits you, you may feel like you are leading a double life. This is a great time to methodically plan for the rest of your life. It is important to know that not having your life in order after 40 and beyond is selfish and isolating. Again, clutter leads to disorganization, which leads to being financially irresponsible, which results in chronic stress and loneliness. If you say you don't care what happens to you, it's my life and screw everyone, you alienate those around you. You need your family and friends, especially when age gets the better of you. I have seen many times when people are mean and defensive, they end up alone later in life and it is very sad. Keep in mind, it's never too late to be happy!

If you are in your 50's, your great-grandmother was probably born around 1895. A woman born at that time could expect to live to about age 45. By the time she was 40, she was an old woman and had lived a complete life. She had given birth and raised her children. She had learned nearly everything she would ever learn. To use the old adage, her best years were behind her. About all she had to look forward to were a few years of declining health ending in death from an illness doctors did not understand and could not cure. As much as modern technology and its benefits are all around us, and can help us, many of our beliefs about aging come from our ancestors and their history.

According to insurance actuaries, if you're 50 today, you still have on average, about 35 years of life to look forward to. Thus you have all the positives your great-grandmother had at your age, yet virtually none of the negatives. Thanks to modern medicine and technology, you can still launch a completely new career, get married, go to college, start a business — virtually anything you want — including having the best sex of your life.

The difference between those days and today are night and day. Many people in their 50s are just beginning to experience the freedom of having no children in the house, or the joys of their first grandchildren, or reaching the pinnacle of their careers, or enjoying time to pursue their hobbies in retirement. At this age, we often pursue renewed vigor and health by taking an interest in fitness, trying out things like a couch-to-5k program to get active... developing or deepening a regular yoga practice... joining a local gym or walking club or sports team to socialize in a fun, fitness-focused environment... biking and hiking and swimming and dancing and mountain climbing and on and on...

"Set a goal and see it through, that's the best confidence booster as we age"

You Create Your Own Reality — At Any Age

Nonetheless, while pursuing our best and healthiest years to come, mourning the loss of your youth is perfectly normal!

Physical changes are inevitable. No matter how hard you work out, how closely you watch your nutrition, you will never look the same as you did at 20. Skin resiliency declines, muscle wasting is inevitable — but let it be said, you will certainly look and feel 100% better if you focus on fitness and nourishing food than if you didn't! Nothing will stave off aging forever, but being healthy lets you enjoy life a lot longer.

Rather than look back on where you were, practice gratitude for where you are, what you have overcome, where you are headed. Create new visions and goals for yourself to achieve, and the

> "As we grow up, we learn that even the one person that wasn't supposed to ever let you down probably will. You will have your heart broken probably more than once and it's harder every time. You'll break hearts too, so remember how it felt when yours was broken. You'll fight with your best friend.
>
> "You'll blame a new love for things an old one did. You'll cry because time is passing too fast, and you'll eventually lose someone you love. So take too many pictures, laugh too much, and love like you've never been hurt because every sixty seconds you spend upset is a minute of happiness you'll never get back. Don't be afraid that your life will end, be afraid that it will never begin."– Anonymous

challenge will fill you with energy and a positive outlook on a day to day basis.

Old flames and lost dreams. This is exactly what it is, over and done with, and for your own sake, it would be healthy to accept this reality and move on. There is a fine line between pursuing lifelong dreams and knowing when you can't do it anymore. It may be time to develop new, more realistic goals for this stage of life.

Don't idolize anyone, especially from the past, not even your past self. Your high school rivals who blossomed then, had their time, now you have yours. You never know who and why people made a great life for themselves, or are living in squalor now. Let go of old crushes, hopes, resentments, and live in the present. It is an incredibly freeing experience to finally do so.

Did you always want to be a prima ballerina as a young girl? An astronaut? A concert pianist? A major league baseball player? These dreams are probably in your past — and there are only a small handful of people who ever achieve these goals in life. Now is the time to regroup, and create new, meaningful goals that will serve you going forward. I always wanted to be an astronaut so I went to the NASA center at Cape Canaveral and learned all about the training, sat in the Mercury capsule — and now I am glad I didn't go into space! Still, I celebrate the memory of my youthful ambition; this year I ran multiple 5k races in honor of the 20th year of the moon landing, and enjoyed the TV shows and museum displays on the historic event that was so meaningful to me.

Taking emotional risks. Get rid of your secrets, they are far worse hidden in your mind then what anyone else will think of them. Find a mentor or a good friend that you trust, and share whatever it is you keep inside that keeps you from moving forward. It is very freeing and you will find a lightness that comes from letting it out, and letting it go.

Self-esteem should increase with age. It isn't always easy to follow the advice of these self-help books that tell you to look in the mirror every day and say, "I am worthy." If you don't believe it, you will never convey it to the outside world. One way to validate your reality is to hang around with people your own age, people you can relate to more easily, rather than trying to stay young by hanging with a crowd that you don't have anything in common with... or who make you feel like you don't quite fit in.

Go back and look at the sidebar in Chapter 2 about the Journal of Compliments, and give it a try. Go for advanced work and try the list of gratitudes as well! Once you have a notebook filled with observations about your days, a written record of all the positive things both within you and surrounding you in your life, it will improve your attitude toward yourself and everyone else.

"The past is gone, the future is uncertain, so treat yourself to the present that is today"

Still, there is a part of everyone's aging process that requires grieving. We mourn the loss of our youth, our physical ease, our hopes for the future. But when you look in the mirror and you see a stranger looking back at you, you are denying who you are right now. This denial will ruin your life, and you have plenty of it left. There is nothing more sad then seeing an older person kicking and scratching to hang on to the past. Change careers; try something else, less taxing, more fun, more meaningful. Seek out a position where you are not judged for being old, but appreciated and valued for your experience and insight. Enjoy who are you are today. Consider moving to a new location to see life in a new and different way.

Get out and about! If you don't want to move, try visiting a different place; maybe visit a city if you live in a rural or suburban area, or visit the country if you live in a busy metropolitan center, or just visit a completely new city or country that you've never been to before, and perhaps always wanted to see. Go on a trip you have dreamed about but never thought you could do. Being away for a week will refresh you. Taking a longer trip will give you a new perspective on how you live, and perhaps how you perceive the world at large.

Taking emotional risks is not exactly a license to live with reckless abandon, but it's certainly inspirational to motivate you to do what you love. At least try out new things to see if something inspires you in a way that you didn't expect or anticipate. When the end is near, be like Sinatra and as the song title says, say you did it "My Way".

"No, that is the great fallacy: the wisdom of old men. They do not grow wise. They grow careful." – Ernest Hemingway

End of Life Care for Loved Ones — and Yourself

While we will address the nitty-gritty of preparing for our advancing years in the next chapter, a few words about it under the topic of relationships as we age is appropriate here. Caring for an aging parent or parents, and the evolution of that lifelong relationship, is delicate and emotionally charged. Lately it seems that all my peers and I talk about are aging parents. We are aging along with our parents, and maybe even grandparents, and we are all trying to muddle through as best we can. It is important to understand that this is inevitable, and it is in your best interest to try to stay calm and accepting throughout the process. I dealt with the illness, decline, and death of both of my parents, and then dealt with the process all over again with my aunt, uncle, cousins, sister-in-law, and mother-in-law. It is never easy, and yes, it reminds us of what lies ahead for us all.

When people age, which hopefully we all will, there reaches a point when you need assistance for at least a few things. If your family member is still mentally sharp, but physically incapacitated, mental stimulation is crucial. If your family member is physically capable but declining mentally, he or she needs to be supervised at all times. These two scenarios take time, patience and money to deal with. It can make you very angry, or frightened, and you may end up taking it out on yourself, or the family member who needs the care, or your immediate circle of close relatives and friends.

It is critical that you start planning for your loved ones and yourself as early as possible, so you're not dealing with challenging circumstances on an emergency basis. It's so much easier to address these issues when they are not at the crisis stage. This is the time to get the help you need. Contact your local hospital, nursing home, or community serves center and find out where you can get a social worker that will assist you in setting up your home, your finances and your psychological well-being for the care of an aging relative. He or she will help you navigate the legalities and expenses related to keeping someone at home, or sending them to a facility.

And be sure to get support for yourself, as well. There is nothing more stressful and upsetting than serving as the main caregiver or organizer of support for an aging parent, spouse, or even for yourself. Parents of special needs children (or adult children) often have to deal with caring for their parents and their children at the same time, and they are truly headed for burnout without support. After discussing the negative health effects of stress, on your fitness, nutrition, sleep, and mental and emotional well-being, be sure to focus on your own health, or you will be no good to anyone else.

Eat well tip
It is very important while providing care for others to ensure that you are taking care of your own health. Like the instructions on the airplane to put on your own oxygen mask before helping those around you — because if you collapse, you can't help anyone! Be sure to pay special attention to your nutrition and hydration. This can go either way: while some people don't eat or drink enough as they worry about their loved ones, other put on extra pounds from stress eating and not tending to their own exercise program. Remember, you are important, too. Take care of yourself, so you can be there for those you love.

As noted above, no matter how much you tend to your own and your family's health, fitness, nutrition, and overall well-being, decline and death are inevitable. The more we embrace this stage of life as part of the pattern of our existence, the less fear and trembling it exerts over us. There are people who can help to plan farewell parties — so much more fun than planning a wake or a funeral, because you get to be there! — for people who are in terminal conditions. This enables them to actually see and say goodbye to their loved ones, while they are still able to do so, and to design the gathering to their own desires.

There are fabulous resources available through AARP and Medicare, and what you learn to help your loved ones will become the basis for a life plan for yourself, as we'll discuss in the next chapter.

Interactive Chapter Review

Relationships As We Age. Who is in your circle today? Spouse? Friends? Pets? Children? Parents? Colleagues? Do they make you feel safe and secure? Do they make you feel good about yourself?

Do you still have toxic people in your life who make you feel bad? What can you do to remove them from your life, or minimize the negative effects?

The Benefits of Family. *What are you relationships like within your family? Have you suffered significant losses or estrangements? Have you created a "family of choice"? Have you made efforts to stay in touch with your family?*

How about friends? Do you have long-term friendships, new friends with whom you share common interests, a few close friends? Have you found ways to get out and make new friends?

Are you in — or would you like to be in — a romantic relationship? Or are you happy on your own? If you are single, have you considered online dating, or how dating "rules" have changed in recent years?

Shared Living Arrangements. *If you are considering moving in with someone — whether as a partner or a roommate — have you established a plan for your finances? How to handle household chores? Are you considerate of each other?*

If you have a big house, are you considering downsizing to a smaller one, single-level, rental apartment or condo? Do finances and health have an impact on this decision, or access to family and friends?

Going It Alone. *If you want to live by yourself, will you have a pet? Do you have family or friends you can check in with regularly to ensure you are well and safe? Do you have resources to help with household repairs? Are there group activities that will keep you from suffering loneliness?*

Have you taken stock of your psychological health and well-being as you age? Have you addressed any long-standing issues? Are you pursuing growth and development on your own, with a counselor, or with a group?

Create Your Own Reality. *While you may be mourning your youth, are you giving yourself new challenges, dreams,* *and goals to strive for? Have you let go of unrealistic or negative youthful ideals? Do you have practices to increase your self-esteem and positive self-regard?*

Have you tried new things in recent years? New foods, new activities, new thoughts, new relationships? Have you considered moving to a new home, or traveling to a new place?

Caregiver Stress. *Are you dealing with organizing or handling end of life care for your aging parents or spouse? Are you seeking out support for yourself during this stressful time? What do you do to help remain calm, so you can continue to help your loved ones?*

Chapter 10
Moving Forward

"Don't be afraid that your life will end, be afraid that it will never begin"

Even a life well lived must come to an end. We are talking about eating well, living well and aging well — not living forever. Immortality is not a reality for us; the only thing we are absolutely certain of in life is that we will eventually die. While some philosophical (or depressive) types may contemplate their death more than others, for many of us, the end of life is seen as a harsh reality that we do not want to face until it happens. Even people with life-threatening diagnoses engage in magical thinking and put off facing the inevitable, hoping for a miracle cure... which may happen, but even that only postpones the final outcome.

We may not know how, and we certainly don't know when, but death will come for us all. While the aim of aging well is to have what is called "reduced morbidity" or a shorter time of living poorly prior to death, not everyone has a smooth transition and your decline could go on for years. It is best to look forward with a cool head, well in advance of when such planning is needed, and to prepare for what we all know is on the horizon for us.

"Do not try to live forever, you will not succeed." – George Bernard Shaw

For everyone else's sake, have your life and finances in good order, and plan for your heirs' financial (and emotional) well-being. If you want to spend all of your money when you are alive, that is your prerogative, but if you don't leave instructions, the government, or someone else other than your spouse and children, can get it — possibly even conniving distant relatives, in-laws, and exes, including those with whom you may have had a falling out — or worse still, con men and crooks who prey upon the elderly, frail, and sick.

There is so much help out there in the world for free, the amount of resources are endless. You just have to reach out and find a plan that works for you and your loved ones.

"A graceful and honorable old age is the childhood of immortality." – Pindar

All the other aspects of aging well that we have been discussing throughout this book will also help our families as well as ourselves: by having our homes in order, they won't have to plow through mountains of belongings and papers (and perhaps come across items or notes or pictures you never wanted them to encounter). If we have advance directives and health care proxies in place, we don't leave them wondering and worrying what we would have wanted them to do. If we take care of our nutrition and fitness and health care, they won't blame themselves (or each other) for not taking better care of us. If we age well, and face our mortality with a positive attitude, we will leave them with happy memories and a wonderful example of how to age with grace, welcoming the next great adventure with the same gusto we have embraced living.

"Recently my family attended a memorial service for a friend who died after a long illness. He was 64 with a youthful soul and a young family. The gravestone only states the day he was born and the day he died. The dash, the time in between, told a story of a life well lived."

Death and Taxes

The old joke says these are the only two things in life which are inevitable — and indeed, managing our finances is one of our mandatory obligations. Develop a relationship with an accountant and get your papers in order. Find out what you need to keep from past income tax returns, and shred the rest of it. Throughout the course of the year, file your papers orderly and give your accountant or bookkeeper the records and receipts on time. If you prepare your own tax returns, you will have everything right where you need it, and in the event you need to go back and find something, the file box should be readily accessible and the paperwork at your fingertips.

If you are adept with technology, get a computer program to manage your finances. We are only moving more and more towards a world where we receive and pay bills electronically, establish and handle our accounts online, and communicate with financial institutions in the same way. Already most banks charge to send you a paper statement rather than simply provide them online, possibly sending you an email notification that it is available. It makes sense to start getting comfortable with this inevitable reality sooner rather than later.

Similarly, most travel arrangements, from airline trips to hotel bookings to cruises, are cheaper to book online than on the phone, and you print out your own tickets and conditions of carriage (or bring them on your smartphone) rather than have them mailed to you. And speaking of travel — if you do start to travel more in your later years, whether you retire or have just earned more vacation time (or perhaps even work while traveling) you will experience the freedom of being able to manage your finances and pay your bills online where ever you are in the world, rather than having someone collect your mail and communicate with you, or write checks to creditors on your behalf while you're on the road.

If you are not comfortable or not capable of managing your money on your own, and you need to pay a fee to an accountant or financial advisor to help you with these matters, then do so. In the event of your death, your loved ones can sort through your papers with a minimum of hassle. You may have an aversion to straightening out your life, but leaving a mess for your heirs will cause them undue stress, on top of the pain of losing your presence in their lives.

While you're at it, write a clear and detailed will so there is no fighting at your funeral or afterwards. Look into living trusts and shared bank accounts so your heirs have access to funds while probate is ongoing. Consult with an experienced trust and estate attorney or accountant to help you establish what you need. Do your best to leave your accounts in an orderly fashion, and prevent more suffering around your loss, which will cause suffering enough for those you love, and who love you and will miss you.

Of course, if you have no children or other family heirs — or even if you do! — you may choose to do what many jokingly (or at least semi-jokingly) call taking "SKI vacations"... that is "Spending our Kids Inheritance"! As noted above, if you prefer to spend your money to the last penny during your lifetime, that is your right. However, many do like to plan for whatever may be left over once they are gone, whether to leave that for family and friends, or as a planned gift to a favorite charity, nonprofit, or educational institution.

"If you're in the luckiest one per cent of humanity, you owe it to the rest of humanity to think about the other 99 percent." – Warren Buffett

Managing Our Finances As We Age

Earning power peaks in the second half of our 40s. Living well also means having the resources to enjoy life and not lose sleep over money or lack of it. Stress over money causes health problems, relationship problems, reduced productivity at work, and clouds your judgment, often making us vulnerable to fraud or "get-rich-quick" schemes (or at least wasting our money on lots of lottery tickets).

We live in a society where we compare ourselves to young tech billionaires and larger-than-life celebrities, which has skewed our perception of what is financial security. Part of feeling content is learning to be satisfied at our financial level and to live within our means.

After 50 it would be a good idea to turn some of your investments into cash on hand. Cash in the bank is not wasted! The reason you worked so hard all these years is to have comfort. The comfort should be yours and yours alone. Working solely to leave money for your children is not to your benefit in old age. Remember, you can always take out a loan for your children's (or grandchildren's) college educations — you cannot take out a loan for your retirement.

At age 60 and beyond, you can start taking assets out of your name. At this point you can gift them to your children, and start a fund that helps them, and if need be, helps you. Again, consult with an experienced tax attorney, estate planner, or accountant about what will work best for your personal situation and your family.

> **"For age is opportunity no less**
> **Than youth itself, though in another dress,**
> **And as the evening twilight fades away**
> **The sky is filled with starts, invisibly by day."**
> **– Henry Wadsworth Longfellow**

Lifestyle Changes

The instructions for how to manage money as we age are often the opposite of what we learned when we were younger. We might have been trying to "dress for success," or "live the lifestyle of the job you want to have, not the one you do," and thus spent more on cars, clothes, residences, vacations, and other expenses, with the hopes that this would attract more wealth into our lives, and make us feel comfortable living at a higher economic level. This is no longer true (if it ever was), and could be downright dangerous to your continued financial well-being. Likewise, your investment mix should be less risky as you move closer to or enter retirement.

> **"It is sad when people live above their means, to**
> **keep up with society, to impress others who don't**
> **care about them – and then end up with nothing"**

The best way to get ahead is to live below your means and not compete with anyone. Living above your means, putting on a show, looking like you have the most on the block only hurts you. It is important as we age that we budget and plan ahead, to make sure our resources will last us the rest of our lives, whether we continue to work or whether we have retired.

On the other hand, if you have been diligent about contributing to your IRA, preparing for your retirement, and your savings are all

Early Signs of Financial Decline in the Elderly

The National Endowment for Financial Education compiled this checklist of early warning signs that may indicate when an older adult's financial competence is declining:
- Reduced attention to details in financial documents
- Decline in everyday math skills

Taking longer to complete everyday financial tasks, such as:
- Prepare bills for mailing Fill out a check register
- File income taxes

Having trouble:
- Identifying an overdue bill that needs attention
- Finding specific details in a bank statement
- Filling out columns of a check register
- Calculating a return on an investment
- Figuring a tip in a restaurant
- Making multiple calculations

Source: National Endowment for Financial Education
By The New York Times

in place, now might be the time to enjoy the fruits of your labors! Whether you retire or not, you can begin to take out money and perhaps take a trip — to another country, another state, or just a new restaurant — and reap the rewards of your focused savings during your younger years.

Perhaps you want to help out your children, grandchildren, or friends, whether paying for college or graduate school, starting a business, or setting up a home. Just make sure you will have enough for yourself and your own needs.

Saving and Investing

Money management experts tell us in order to have retirement money we should diligently save 10% of our income throughout our working lives. If you are not earning much right now, or this seems impossible with your current expenses, how about starting out small? Save a dollar a day, at the end of the year you will have 365 dollars to do whatever you want with. If you can save 5 dollars a day, then at the end of the year, you will have $1825.00. You can start an investment account, use it for an unexpected emergency, or a reward yourself with a vacation. Banks offer many "automatic" savings programs that set aside a certain amount of money every week or every paycheck, to ensure that your nest egg will grow.

You may have a pension or other defined benefit plan where you work, and if you work for a company that matches IRA contributions up to a certain amount you should aim to put aside that amount every year you are working. The compounding interest will add up fast, even if you start in your later years, and you put in pre-tax dollars now, and withdraw them later when you will presumably be in a lower tax bracket.

If you anticipate continuing to have a higher tax rate even after retirement, consider opening a Roth IRA which lets you put in after-tax money and then withdraw it after age 59 with no tax penalty whatsoever. While you must start taking withdrawals from traditional IRAs by age 70, there are no distribution requirements for Roth IRAs, so they can continue to grow tax-free, and can be left to heirs who can also take tax-free distributions from the account. Furthermore, if you start your Roth IRA when you are younger, you can take distributions once your account is 5 years old with no penalty; you can't do that with a traditional IRA. Talk with your financial planner to see what works best for your situation.

You may also come into money as you age, as the previous generation passes on and you come into an inheritance. This is a time to seek financial assistance and guidance, particularly if you have not managed a large estate before. Help with investing, saving, and preparing for your own future are critical, so you don't treat this as a "windfall" and rush out to spend this money without thinking.

When we were younger, we were taught to invest money in real estate and the stock market, that the tiny interest earned on savings in the bank meant we were effectively wasting our money. However, as we age, less is more in the way of investments, especially risky ones. Being liquid and having cash on hand will serve you better than having it tied up in volatile stocks or hard-to-sell real estate. The less you gamble with your money, both in business and recreationally, the less susceptible you are to market swings. Stay liquid after 60 and stick to your plan for later in life.

Gambling

And speaking of gambling: along with late-onset alcoholism, excessive gambling is one of the dangers for retired, isolated adults. Many social settings involve certain aspects of gambling, such as bingo or penny-ante poker, sports betting or lottery pools. It is easy to move from these safe havens with friends to commercial gambling establishments. Casinos are set up to be inviting and entertaining sites, often offering free drinks as well to help you lose your inhibition, caution, and common sense.

You may be tempted to "keep up" with friends or the people around you, who may have more money to play with, and get yourself into trouble unintentionally. You might even have friends who are professional poker or blackjack players, and know all the rules to "beat the house." This may look easy, but it takes a lot of time and practice, and they know to avoid the games with the worst odds, especially slot machines. And even professionals can have big losses.

Be careful not to overspend — no matter how much money you may or may not have — on games of chance, which are always run with a huge advantage to the house. While you may have that one-in-a-million chance to win the lottery, the card game, the slot machine — those "one-armed bandits" got their name for a good reason: they are there to steal your money. Don't let yourself be led down this lonely road. A good rule of thumb is to spend no more on gambling than you would on a night out at a restaurant and the theatre — with the chance of winning back the cost of your ticket and your meal. But that's it!

Insurance

Make sure your insurance policies are in place and current. In addition to basic health insurance, you will want disability, long-term care, homeowners, and life insurance. In the event you have a catastrophic illness or event, you need to be prepared. More families and individuals can be wiped out financially by a medical crisis (stroke, heart attack, cancer) or home disaster (fire, flood, collapse) than any other situation. Make sure your loved ones know where to find your policies, or how to contact your insurance agent. If you travel, be sure to get trip insurance since your health insurance may not cover you out of your area. Also, you want to be covered for any losses, and especially in case you need medical evacuation.

Social service policies have made a huge change in overall poverty rates among the elderly: in 1966, 29 percent of people over age 65 lived below the poverty line, while in 2014 that had decreased to just 10 percent. (*Federal Interagency Forum on Aging: 2016 — Older Americans Key Indicators of Well-Being*) However, do not count on "the system" to take care of you! Most government support programs are only for those who have virtually no income or assets; you would have to divest yourself of your home and your life savings before these benefits become available. It is very difficult to transfer assets to other family members so that you can access these programs. (*See "End of Life Planning" below for more details on insurance policies it is good idea to have in place, for peace of mind and to prevent placing unnecessary financial burdens on your family.*)

Protect Yourself From Fraud

There are a few simple steps in which you can take to prevent fraudulent activity on your bank accounts, credit cards, and protect your investments. Start by consolidating your accounts as you age; it is easier to manage you financial life if you keep it simple. While you don't want to have "all your eggs in one basket," you can still diversify your investments without having a dozen separate accounts — or worse, a dozen separate credit cards. Make it simpler to track your saving and spending to ensure that you don't miss any fraudulent activity.

We often hear how fraud is an inside job, at the bank, the stores we frequent, and sometimes even our friends and family. If it is difficult for you to manage, at least give the appearance that you are diligent about knowing your account balances and activities. I always check my receipts to see if I have been charged properly, and even if I don't think I need the receipt I take it with me. This gives the impression to anyone that might be watching that you are "with it" and on top of your finances, and thus you will be a less likely target for fraud.

If you get any aggressive sales calls, or threatening calls from individuals claiming to be with a utility company or tax authority, don't get rattled, and certainly don't agree quickly to send money online, by wire transfer, or by using prepaid gift cards. Get their contact information, hang up, and check the phone number or email with the official government website. If you suspect a scammer is in action, report them to the police, the FBI, or the Better Business Bureau. You may save someone else from being taken advantage of.

"To find joy in work is to discover the fountain of youth." – Pearl S. Buck

Work and Retirement

Many older people have delayed retirement; 42 percent of people over age 65 are either working full or part-time. This often can be a challenge, since older people are not given an equal chance for paid employment. In corporate downsizings and mergers, the first to go are the older workers, even though it is now illegal to force retirement. In job seeking, older workers are viewed as posing liabilities, being likely to retire soon or increase medical costs while contributing only a few years to the company's bottom line.

The fact is, millions of older people are ready, willing and able to work. Employers who focus on the retention and recruitment of older employees find that they meet or exceed expectations, and bring valuable insight and experience to the table. Many older workers enjoy finding a second (or sixth!) career during the time previous generations would have retired. Some may choose to move from a high-pressure business environment to a community service organization, perhaps earning a lower salary but taking home much higher personal rewards.

"Employers who focus on the retention and recruitment of older employees find that they meet or exceed expectations"

If you're planning to stop working, make it a rewarding time. According to a landmark Harvard University study of aging, that means replacing the human contact you enjoyed with co-workers by spending time with new friends, rediscovering how to play, pursuing a creative outlet, and continually learning new things. And as noted above, you will want to save money to prepare for this time when your income will be reduced once you stop working.

"Old age hath yet his honour and his toil." – Tennyson

To ensure that your savings, and any pension or Social Security income will last, step away from the credit cards, checkbooks, and savings accounts. There's no need to buy every new gadget; chances are you need so much less that what you already have. Channel your energy into social causes that are near and dear to you, rather than spending money on pricey outings or "retail therapy." Learn the joys of volunteerism and making a difference by contributing your time and expertise to serve others. Rediscover the library, take advantage of cultural offerings during the day at reduced prices for students and seniors, including movies, plays, music and dance concerts, especially if you are in an urban area or a college town.

"The harvest of old age is the recollection and abundance of blessings previously secured." – Cicero

Get outdoors, visit local parks and gardens, become familiar with your natural surroundings. It doesn't cost anything to take a walk in the park, alone or with friends. Getting closer to nature is a very therapeutic experience. It will increase environmental awareness and your consciousness of and connectedness to the larger world around you. Join a local walking group — these are often organized through senior centers and YMCA/YMHAs — and enjoy the double benefit of being in nature and party of a community. And you'll begin to create a new social network of other people who are interested in healthy aging, appreciating nature, and the simpler things in life.

> **"There is a fountain of youth: it is your mind, your talents, the creativity you bring to your life and the lives of people you love. When you learn to tap this source, you will truly have defeated age." - Sophia Loren**

Become Tech Savvy

Technology has moved so fast and continues to do so. The world has changed so rapidly and drastically, that the nature of how we communicate has changed as well. Being aware of changes and how to integrate them into your life is an ongoing process. This means keeping up with the technology that will keep your personal information safe from exposure and fraud, and keep you "in the loop" on discussions of new technology as it arrives in our lives. Some great ways to get yourself up to speed is taking an adult education class at a local library, community college, or an online course that is easy to follow.

I consider myself a tech laggard, but even I have learned how to use technology to my advantage. I enjoy reading books and magazines in the traditional way, but if I am traveling I will use a tablet or e-reader... browse and shopping online... tracking my steps with my GPS watch... handling banking and bill paying electronically... watching movies and TV shows on my phone... communicating with friends and getting the latest news online

Steve Greenberg, CEO of ThinClient Computing in Scottsdale, AZ recommends the following:

"Everyone is at a different level of technical understanding and no one can know it all. What is important is to always keep learning something new. Don't try to take on more than you feel you can handle, but every day try to learn something new. Just one small new piece of information, understanding or insight every day adds up to huge returns over even a small amount of time.

"As far as tech goes, take one thing at a time that perhaps you don't understand and work on it. Maybe it is how to do formatting in a Word document, how to compare prices on the Internet, how to use video conferencing, texting, email or any other tool that you are not currently comfortable with. The time is takes to learn how to do it will invigorate your mind and possibly open you up to highly valuable new experiences."

through social media, with my kids through texts and instant messaging, with my husband and clients via email — and yet I make sure to still get together with friends in person, visit favorite local stores, attend live theatre, read hardcover or paperback books, enjoy hard-copy printed magazines and newspapers, and generally live an off-line life.

You have surely noticed how technology has dramatically affected our relationships and social skills. People now seem to feel that they have no need to be polite and considerate, especially if all of our day-to-day transactions are happening online. Younger service staff tends to be less attentive to older, less tech savvy customers in all industries, and we may feel belittled or ignored when we try to get customer service attention in many areas.

Unfortunately, young adults now seem to lack the vocabulary, patience and demeanor to be kind to an older person, who may not know the latest and greatest trends. Many of us feel we are constantly being dismissed and misunderstood. It is generational, and you don't have to join that club to be heard. Let us all aim to be role models, and treat others as we would like to be treated! We can share our experience of how to treat each other with kindness, politeness, and respect, and hope that the younger folk will follow are example.

Charitable Giving and Volunteerism

Many people give to charity because they feel a responsibility to take care of others less fortunate. This includes giving money, volunteering your time, and/or contributing other resources. The first question you have to ask yourself is: can I afford to give away my money, time, and resources? Then you have to ask yourself some harder questions, and really answer them honestly: What is your personal motivation for giving? Do you see it as an opportunity to advance professionally? Are you trying to buy status in your community?

"Wherever you turn, you can find someone who needs you. Even if it is a little thing, do something for which there is no pay but the privilege of doing it. Remember, you don't live in the world all of your own." – Albert Schweitzer

Don't give away money until your own financial house is in order. Many people give out of guilt, or to look good in front of others, rather than because they genuinely wish — and have the means — to help others. If charitable giving is at the expense of your own well-being, stop giving and start saving. This is in no way intended for you to become selfish, but to get you grounded. If you have the means to do so, research and connect with institutions with which you have a heartfelt affinity, and support them with financial contributions, volunteer your time, or in-kind donations as appropriate for you.

Volunteering can sometimes lead to paid work, but for the most part in measuring success, our society simply doesn't count unpaid work as part of the equation for measuring contribution to society. We labor under society's assumption is that those who work for pay are pulling their own weight, while those who do not are a burden. Yet, in the larger sense, older people are productive and contribute to society. Many of us still work for pay, and older people — whether working or retired — work as volunteers in religious organizations, hospitals, schools, or charities, and others provide informal aid to family members, friends, neighbors, students, and young people.

"Pay it forward — Providing for someone in need, with no expectation of anything in return, is the utmost form of giving"

If you are in a position to do so, look into the many opportunities for living trusts administered by various charitable organizations, nonprofit groups and educational institutions. These may allow you to donate funds which will be managed to generate income during your lifetime, and then pass to your selected charity upon your death. These groups do this to ensure they will receive large bequests, but in the meantime you benefit by having your money managed by a large organization that will have more financial "clout" and result in better income than simply investing on your own.

You may also consider naming certain beloved charities in your will as recipients of specific bequests to make sure that your money goes where you want it to. Perhaps you want to endow a scholarship at your school or one of your children's schools, or make a large contribution to your church or synagogue, or donate cash or a valuable gift of artwork or furnishings to a social organization that you believe in and have supported while you were alive. This is a wonderful way to leave a legacy of who you were — however, as noted above, make sure that you have provided for yourself and your family before you start making plans for charitable donations. As the saying goes: Charity begins at home.

"The elders in our society are now the role models for the younger generations that are coming of age. This is a chance to give back and teach our children to show up for life and be present every day"

Exercise Your Mind

People who read, play board games, do crossword puzzles and play musical instruments in their 70s have a lower risk of developing dementia. Physical exercise also helps. Women who walk during their 60s are significantly less likely to show mental decline in their 70s. Blood flow to the brain, caused by activity, helps mental function.

With the number of Americans afflicted with Alzheimer's disease projected to triple to nearly 14 million by 2050, research on the devastating brain disorder is taking on new urgency. Scores of experiments are being launched that might yield better diagnosis, prevention and treatment in five to 10 years. There are dozens of new "anti-aging" websites that provide interactive content to keep your brain engaged and active.

"For the unlearned, old age is winter; for the learned, it is the season of the harvest." – Hasidic saying

Many great universities offer free courses online for seniors, and you may even choose to pursue a degree at a local institution. Why not? You are never too old to learn, or to pursue dreams you think may have passed you by. I have a friend who went to med school in his 40s and finally fulfilled his lifelong dream to be a physician, following in the footsteps of his parents, albeit two decades later than most people who go down this career path.

In the meantime, keep thinking, keep moving, and continue to pursue your interests, old and new. Think about "older people" you knew when you were younger: they seemed to get stiff mentally as well as physically, "stuck in their ways," holding onto old thoughts and habits of thinking without allowing any new opinions or views to sway their long-established beliefs. It seemed as if they were set in stone. For those of us who want to live well and age well, learning new information, exploring new ideas, being open to new approaches, engaging in spirited debate, all helps to keep us young.

"Live as if you were to die tomorrow. Learn as if you were to live forever." – Mahatma Gandhi

A Centered Life

Studies show that organized religion and faith-based groups seem to provide happiness for seniors. Attending religious services may not make us happier, but observing holidays as part of religious activity tends to raise our spirits when in a communal setting. This has important implications for people facing the emotional and physical trials that can come with aging. There is something to be said for the bonds that families develop by having religious rituals and holidays. Families are more likely to be closer and spend time together by celebrating and worshipping together. If religion is not your thing, trying group activities of any sort will help. You will inevitably find a like-minded person to pal around and share good times with.

If there is anything you need to say to someone, perhaps an apology or just letting them know they are loved, write it down, maybe with pictures, and send that letter! If you are having a hard time with it, ask someone to help you compose the piece for you. It would be wonderful to let that person know after all you have been through, and after you are gone, that he or she was loved, admired, forgiven and valued. For your own mental well-being, if that person is already beyond reach, you could still write the letter for yourself.

Lastly, know in your heart that all human beings on this planet did the best they could at every moment of their lives. When we get to our final days and reflect on how we lived, know that your life has value and you have made a unique, everlasting contribution to the world.

"In the end, it's not the years in your life that count. It's the life in your years." – Abraham Lincoln

Organized Religion & Spirituality

Organized religion can be a starting point, but spirituality is what will center you. By incorporating spirituality into your life, you don't have to change your whole life, or lifestyle. You can take what you need and leave the rest! There is a very happy medium between being totally religious and being totally secular, because that division is an artificial one. Rather than boxing people into religious or secular, know that there is a wide spectrum of beliefs and observances out there, and only you can decide what works best for you. Don't be afraid to be unconventional, it is an individual choice.

This isn't a plug for any one religion. Just becoming aware of the greater forces around you is enlightening. It is very challenging for all of us is to live and grow in that gray area of not knowing where we came from or where we are going. It can be comforting to share your spiritual experiences with a community of like-minded individuals, and have a place to go every day, or every week, or even once a year and feel a sense of belonging.

"A human being would certainly not grow to be 70 or 80 years old if this longevity had no meaning for the species to which he belongs. The afternoon of human life must also have a significance of its own and cannot be merely a pitiful appendage to life's morning." – Carl Jung

Don't be afraid to reach beyond your comfort zone, visit a worship or prayer service with a friend who belongs to a different congregation or religion, read books on meditation or other spiritual practice. Many people regard physical activity as a kind of "moving meditation," where they have quiet time to focus their thoughts, whether running, swimming, biking, practicing martial arts or yoga, or engaging in some other sweat-inducing physical sport. They gain the benefit of both personal growth and improved physical fitness — and as noted above, the blood flow to the brain and positive endorphins lead to improved mood and outlook on life.

The Importance of Community

Remember the section in Chapter 1 on "Blue Zones" back in the beginning of this book? The importance of being part of a supportive community, family, and society cannot be overstated. Many have theorized that the positive impact of religious or spiritual involvement is not the worship practice itself, but rather being part of a group.

This means you have people with similar interests and beliefs to offer guidance and help you cope with major life transitions — going to school, getting married, having children and grandchildren (and having them go to school), coping with medical crises or financial setbacks, adjusting to aging and life changes, the loss of loved ones, and preparing for death. It's possible that it's not so much the prayer as the potluck that saves us, so even if you feel like you don't have a religious bone in your body, see if you can find a supportive community to be a part of, it may help you to live longer.

"If there is one thing I've learned in my years on this planet, it's that the happiest and most fulfilled people are those who devoted themselves to something bigger and more profound than merely their own self-interest." – John Glenn

Assisted Living

As we age, we also want to think about our housing and residential care. Do we want to remain in our current home? Do we have family and friends who can care for us in case of emergency or gradual health decline, or do we have the financial wherewithal to cover round-the-clock in-home nursing care?

Many people look at the options for 55+ living communities, where there is a built in age-related community, a clubhouse, and planned activities that continue to keep us engaged and socially active. We may also consider moving to a smaller and more manageable rental apartment or condo rather than having to keep up with roof repairs, lawn maintenance, and other demands of home ownership. Changing from a multi-level home that require us to go up and down stairs to a split-level or ranch-style home also reduces the incidence of injuries due to trips and falls.

> **"Why should I fear death?**
> **If I am, then death is not.**
> **If Death is, then I am not.**
> **Why should I fear that which can only**
> **exist when I do not?"– Epicurus**

There are also assisted living facilities, where we can pay full freight for a set number of years, living completely independently within a planned community. Then, if our health declines or we begin to suffer from various medical issues, including the onset of dementia, there are increasing levels of care, from assistance with daily housekeeping and personal issues, to full memory treatments, that are included at the same price.

Look back at Chapter 9, about living situations as we age, for some of the various options you may consider, whether you are in a relationship, longtime or newly single, if you have family nearby or none. It is worthwhile to consider all of these different approaches well in advance of needing to change your residence, so that you can plan for it calmly, rather than being forced into a situation last minute.

End of life planning

Do you want to be buried, cremated, frozen in a cryo-tube, turned into a sea rock? Do you want your ashes scattered in the backyard, at sea, in Kathmandu? Put it in writing, give or send it to a trustworthy family member, and when you die, your wishes will be granted. You will also want to have a living will and health care proxy, so that if you are disabled, a trusted friend or family member will carry out your wishes on your behalf.

No heroic measures? Keep me on life support as long as possible? Whatever it is, put it in writing in a legal document. It's difficult to predict when health problems might leave you unable to make decisions about yourself. Take steps early to clarify your wishes about life-sustaining medical treatment. Completing an advance directive such as a living will can do this.

Here is a breakdown of what you will need you need to ensure your end of life wishes are fulfilled. You can also get more detailed information about this process through your health plan, lawyer or senior advocacy groups.

Health, Disability, & Long-Term Care Insurance

Hopefully you have some health insurance that will help you with the basics. Most of us are not eligible for Medicare until we reach retirement age, or 65. Disability insurance is also a good idea, since there is very little coverage for us if we lose the ability to generate income from work. Worker's Compensation can help if we are injured on the job, and Medicaid may provide some assistance for those at the bottom of the economic ladder, but for the most part we have to prepare to take care of ourselves — or become (unwanted and potentially resented) burdens on our families and loved ones.

Both private insurance and Medicare cover only short-term medical care, so it is important to think ahead about long-term care that we may need in later years. The older you are when you buy long-term care insurance the more expensive it will be. The best time to invest in long-term care is when you are young and healthy. I started my policy in my 40s and so my premiums are still low. Consult an insurance expert and see what plans will work for you.

Advance Directives

Advance directives are the documents you use to describe in detail the medical care you wish to receive in the event you are incapacitated and unable to make your wishes known, especially due to an unexpected event. There is the mistaken assumption that advance directives are only for the elderly or very ill people. The reality is that the younger you are when you put this in place, the better.

These documents in no way take away your rights as long as you are able to make your own decisions. It will allow you to choose the person you would like to have in charge of your health care, and this person will legally become your health care agent, or proxy. Make sure whatever documents you fill out are distributed to more than one person, so there will be no questions if and when the time comes. In the event that you recover from a catastrophic illness or accident, you can redirect your wishes orally and that will take precedence over your written wishes.

A health care power of attorney is a legally binding document that states who you want as your health care agent, also known as a health care proxy. This person will be assigned to fulfilling your wishes when you cannot. In the event that you don't have an assigned agent, a relative or court appointed guardian can make whatever decisions they see fit and there is no recourse. If your family doesn't know what you want, there could be a delay in your treatments or no treatment, ending in disastrous consequences.

DNR (Do Not Resuscitate) or "Heroic Measures"

This is a document that is included in your chart at the hospital or your home in case you go into distress that requires extreme measures to keep you alive. Some life-saving techniques can also be harmful to a very frail person, so it should be carefully considered if you want all measures taken to save your life. Unofficially, hospitals do tend to treat younger people first, so it is very important if you want to be resuscitated at all costs make your wishes known.

Likewise, if you don't want to have what are called "heroic measures" taken to maintain your respiration and heartbeat if there is no measurable brain activity, and simply wish to have palliative or hospice care to reduce pain, it is very important to have a legal document that states this is your wish. If you have religious strictures on certain medical procedures, such as blood transfusions, organ transplants, and so on, this should be made clear as well, since otherwise hospitals have to follow specific protocols.

Living Will

Living wills are legal documents in which you spell out the type of care you wish to receive in catastrophic situations where you may be unconscious or unable to manage your own care. A great source for designing your own living will is the National Hospice and Palliative Care Organization. They have state-specific advance directives that you can obtain online for free: www.caringinfo.org/AdvanceDirectives. You have the option of updating these as often as you wish, so that they are always current.

Living wills often include the designation of a Health Care Proxy or Medical Power of Attorney. This lets you give someone else the authority to make medical decisions on your behalf in case you are incapacitated, unable to express your own wishes, or otherwise oversee and handle your own health care arrangements.

These legal documents are particularly important if you are not in a traditional legal marriage where your spouse can be assumed to be in charge of these matters — or if you prefer to have someone else handle such decisions, if there is concern that your spouse would be too upset by your condition, or possibly similarly incapacitated if you were in an accident while traveling together.

"Death waits for no one"

Wills and Trusts

As noted above under Finances, write out a clear and detailed will to ensure that your possessions and investments and savings go to the person or persons you want to receive them. The estates of people who die intestate, or without a will, are governed by rules that are specific to each state, and usually will divide up your estate between various family members, whether you want them to receive anything or not. Similar to a health care power of attorney, you can assign a financial power of attorney, giving someone the authority to make financial decisions for you in case you are incapacitated and unable to manage your own affairs.

You may wish to consult with an attorney if your will is at all complicated or you have a large estate, in order to maximize the amount that you can leave to your heirs, if there are family conflicts and you fear that people may challenge your will, to minimize taxes, or if you have multiple bequests to outside organizations and unrelated individuals. If your will and family situation is fairly simply, you can probably just use a template for a will that you can find online. Make sure that you sign it with witnesses and have it notarized, and stored in a safe place.

If you have a large estate, or if you want to save your heirs from having to wait until the estate goes through probate before they can access your assets, you may consider establishing a living trust with both you and your heirs listed as trustees. That way, when you're gone they can still manage the assets without having to wait. You can also assign real estate, IRA accounts, and life insurance policies outside of your will, in order to provide access to money faster.

Be sure to choose someone whom you trust and who has the ability to remain level-headed upon your demise to handle your estate. Whoever you name as your executor/executrix will have to obtain multiple copies of letters testamentary, death certificates, and more in order to handle the details of settling your estate, such as paying off any outstanding debts, fulfilling specific bequests and other directives in your will, and so on.

Likewise, if you are named as the executor for someone's will — be that a parent, spouse, significant other, friend, or other relative — you will be acting as the fiduciary agent for that estate, so take a deep breath, schedule a time for crying, mourning, and grieving, and get down to the business that you have been entrusted to handle for your loved one. It helps to keep a notebook so you can track all activities related to the management of the estate: who you call to ask for help, what documents you have requested and when they are received, any services that you request or hire, and the amount of time you spend managing this all. Large estates often direct that executors should be compensated for their time, as well as reimbursing any out-of-pocket expenses you may have to cover while awaiting access to estate funds.

> For everything there is a season, and a time for every purpose under heaven: a time to be born, and a time to die; a time to plant, and a time to pluck up that which is planted; a time to kill, and a time to heal; a time to break down, and a time to build up; a time to weep, and a time to laugh; a time to mourn, and a time to dance; a time to cast away stones, and a time to gather stones together; a time to embrace, and a time to refrain from embracing; a time to seek, and a time to lose; a time to keep, and a time to cast away; a time to rend, and a time to sew; a time to keep silence, and a time to speak; a time to love, and a time to hate; a time for war, and a time for peace. — Ecclesiastes 3:1–8

None of this is easy, and you (or your loved ones) are suffering the pain of loss of the person who has passed on. Be sure to obtain support for yourself — or encourage your heirs to do so — so that you can attend to your responsibilities with care and attention.

"Aging is not a disease but a culmination of all that we have done — right or wrong"

Funerals and "Living Funerals"

If you belong to a religious denomination, this may be handled by your house of worship, and follow a proscribed plan. You can always provide specific wishes or directions for your services to your heirs in your will — whether you want to be cremated or have an open casket, what you want to wear, where the services should be held, etc. For those who do not have a specific affiliation, planning is more open, and you can ask your friends or family to remember you in the way you see best.

Some people — especially those who are living with life-threatening illnesses — often plan a "living funeral" so they can be there for the event! Rather than think about all their friends and family coming together once they are gone, they invite them all to a party while they are still alive, to celebrate and "remember" you before you depart. Do an internet search for "living funeral" to see some ideas.

Interactive Chapter Review

No One Lives Forever. Do you think about death? Often? Sometimes? Rarely? Never? Are you organized, and your finances in order, to help your family cope after you are gone?

Death and Taxes. Do you have an accountant, bookkeeper, financial planner, tax attorney? Do you manage your finances yourself or hire someone to do it for you/with you? Are you able to handle your finances on the computer, pay bills and manage your accounts online?

Do you have a will written so your money goes to who you want it to? Or are you planning to spend all of your money before you die (SKI vacations)? Have you considered leaving money to a favorite charity, nonprofit, or educational institution?

Managing Finances As We Age. Do you still stress out over money problems? Does it cause issues for your health, relationships, sleep? Are you an easy mark for "get-rich-quick" schemes? Are you disappointed with your financial state?

Do you compare yourself to young billionaires? Or are you contented with where you are and what you have? Are you able to leave within your means, or do you always want more?

Saving and Investing. At 50, did you (or will you) change your investment mix so that you have more cash on hand and fewer risky investments? Remember, you can take out a loan for education, but not for retirement! Will you take (or have you taken) assets out of your name when you reach 60?

Lifestyle Changes. *What lifestyle changes have you experienced or do you anticipate as you age? Did you seek more status through spending and showing off, and is that starting to cut back?*

Are you budgeting and planning ahead for changes in income as you age? Or are you finally starting to enjoy taking out of the long-term savings that you have been contributing to all your life?

Have you set up an automatic savings account, or do you set aside a certain amount every week or every month? Have you established a traditional or Roth IRA and make regular contributions?

If you have investments, have you changed your asset mix into more liquidity and less risk? Have you reduced the amount of your net worth that is tied up in real estate?

Gambling. *Do you avoid gambling and games of chance, or if you enjoy these are you careful to stay on budget and not go beyond your means? Do you compare the costs of a night of gambling to a night at dinner and the theatre, or do you use another method to rein in spending?*

Insurance. *Do you have needed insurance policies in place, including health, disability, long-term care, homeowners, life insurance? Do you know anyone who has been wiped out by a catastrophic illness or home loss? Do you think that "the system" will take care of you in a crisis?*

Fraud Prevention. *What steps do you take to protect yourself from fraud? Have you begun to consolidate your accounts to make it easier to track suspicious activity? Do you present as someone who is "with it" and on top of financial transactions in public, taking and reading receipts? Have you ever received any aggressive or threatening calls asking for money? How did you deal with them?*

Work and Retirement. *Are you planning (or hoping) to keep working, or do you plan to retire? Will you continue in the same career, or try out a new field? Do you anticipate earning at the same level you have in the past, or will you have to take a pay cut?*

If you are going to retire, what will you do to fill your days? Have you joined any new organizations, or are you pursuing activities on your own? Will you control spending by enjoying free or low-costs activities for seniors and retirees? How about increasing your physical activity and getting out into nature?

Becoming Tech Savvy. *Are you already tech savvy, or is this something you really want to do? What aspects of modern technology would you like to be more familiar and comfortable with to improve your life on a daily basis?*

Do you read books, watch movies and TV, browse and shop online? Do you communicate with friends, family, colleagues, clients, children, grandchildren via email, text, instant messages, social media? What "real life" activities do you enjoy as well?

Have you noticed that technology has diminished our customer service and human interaction skills, especially for younger people? Have you ever felt belittled for being less tech savvy than others? Do you try to maintain a positive and friendly demeanor, even when people may act in an inconsiderate fashion?

Charitable Giving and Volunteerism. *Do you give to charities, volunteer your time, or donate goods? Why? Do you have a strong affinity for the organization, like helping others, or are you just trying to get a tax deduction, keep up with or look good in front of others, or seeking professional advancement or social connections? Do you have the means to do so, or should you start by getting your own house in order?*

Have you considered setting up a living trust with a favorite charity as the beneficiary, or leaving a specific bequest to a nonprofit organization or educational institution?

Mental Exercise. What do you do to keep your mind active and engaged? Do you continue to work professionally? Do you read, play board games, do crossword puzzles, sing in a choir, play a musical instrument? Are you physically active to keep your brain healthy? Are you concerned about possible dementia or Alzheimer's disease? Are there other anti-aging programs that you follow? What do you think helps to keep you feeling and thinking young?

Religion and Spirituality. Are you a member of any organized religion or faith-based group? Do you observe holidays with family and friends, or enjoy other group activities? Do you share your concerns and joys with this community?

Have you let go of past resentments or anger? Have you made peace, apologized, owned up to wrongs you may have done in the past? Have you tried writing a letter expressing your feelings to someone you have hurt — or who has hurt you — whether you are able to send it or not?

Do you enjoy spiritual practice, whether through organized groups or on your own, in prayer, meditation, contemplation, or "moving meditation" through deeply engaged physical activity? Do you enjoy thinking and wondering about things beyond the visible? Are you open-minded to other people's religious and spiritual practices?

Whether or not you are involved in a religious society, do you enjoy being part of a supportive community? What interests do you share? How have you found being part of a group to help you through difficult times, or how have you helped others who are in the group with your own life experience?

Housing Concerns. Have you considered changing your living situation, whether now or in the future? Have you planned for what to do when you are no longer able to take care of yourself? Will you want to stay in your home, move to a smaller home or planned community, or look into an assisted living facility?

End-of-life Planning. Have you specified in your will how you want your remains to be handled? Do you have legal documents that ensure that someone is in place to handle life-sustaining medical treatment or DNR orders? Is your insurance in place to cover costs? Do you have a will or trust that will distribute your assets to those you want to receive them (and protect it from those you do not)?

Is your funeral or memorial service prescribed by your religious faith? Have you specified what kind of service you would like to be held in your memory? Have you considered hosting a "living funeral" so you can be there to enjoy seeing all of your loved ones come together while you are still alive, rather than after you are dead?

Epilogue

As I was writing this book — from the initial thoughts to putting notes down on paper, gathering information by reading and researching and observing the world around me — I went to friends, family, and experts in their respective fields for feedback, to learn and embrace what it is that you the reader would want to know, and what would speak to you on a deep level about getting old. My hope is after reading this book, that you will not be inclined to spend your later years chasing "anti-aging" schemes to no avail.

I just looked inside myself and thought, what do I need to feel good about going forward in life? "Acceptance" is what always seems to be the answer. What I discovered is that my deepest regrets are the opportunities that I passed by due to fear and insecurity, mostly based on what others would have me believe about myself, rather than trusting my own instincts and going after what I wanted, even if it was not the popular choice.

It never ceases to amaze me that I am still awed by nature's inherent beauty, art, science and technology, people doing amazing things at all ages, and yet deeply connected to my past which was a much simpler time in history. My hope is that it is the same for you. To feel excited about the rest of your life, by staying in the reality of the present, always remember to "**Stay in today,**" value what you have learned, and look for ways to make your future and everyone's around you brighter.

Now in my 50s, I have come to rely 100 percent on myself, I trust myself and I can make decisions with the utmost confidence. Give it a try, you will be surprised at how easily it all comes together. I don't have all the answers and I cannot make anyone else's life better, but if you picked up a few good tips from this book, I will consider this a success for all of us!

My hope is that *Eat Well, Live Well, Age Well* gives you insights to help you improve your life, develop or support positive habits of action and thought, and will continue to be a source of information, inspiration, and even comfort when you feel you are slipping back into old, bad behaviors. My goal is for this book to be a guide at your fingertips, to help you get what you need to achieve physical and emotional wellness. We all want to be happy, healthy and at peace with our decisions. If you are impaired, on a budget, or in an emotional funk, know that there are always ways to improve your life by just reaching out to another person, or tapping into the resources referenced throughout this book.

In closing, I want to say that all of life is a journey to be enjoyed. A journey that is different for all of us, but remarkable similar when it comes down to looking forward towards the rest of our lives.

Happiness and health to you always!

Patricia Greenberg

Questions to Ponder

Remember, there are no right or wrong answers to any of these questions. They are for you to ponder, and your own responses may change from before to after you read this book, and as you make adjustments in your own life.

These are questions I enjoy asking myself on a regular basis, as a checkpoint to see how I'm doing, if I'm continuing to grow and develop emotionally, or if I'm slipping back into less productive ways of reacting to the world around me. I hope you find them useful, too.

How old are you? (What is your biological age in years)

_____

_____

How old do you feel? (What is your chronological age)

_____

_____

How old do you wish you were?

_____

_____

How old do others perceive you to be?

_____

_____

Are you comfortable with your age?

_____

_____

Are you comfortable with the aging process?

_____

_____

How do you like your appearance at this point in your life?

_____

_____

When did you notice the changes of age setting in?

_____

_____

Do you feel that you are treated differently now than when you were younger?

_____

_____

Are you happy?

_____

_____

What is the most extraordinary thing you have seen in your lifetime?

_____

_____

What world event in your lifetime had the most profound impact on you?

_____

_____

What is the most daring thing you have ever done?

_____

_____

Do you have any regrets?

_____

_____

How do you deal with regret?

_____

_____

What is one of your lifelong dreams?

_____

_____

Have you fulfilled it?

_____

_____

How would you rate your physical health?

_____

_____

How is your memory?

_____

_____

What is the highest education level you have completed?

_____

_____

Do you continue to study and learn?

_____

_____

Do you feel that your ethnic background affects your outlook on life?

_____

_____

On a typical day, about how many hours do you sleep?

_____

_____

What are your Exercise Habits?

_____

_____

What are your Hobbies?

_____

_____

How often do you visit with family and friends?

_____

_____

How do you deal with tragedy?

_____

_____

Are you single? How long have you been married/ coupled?

_____

_____

Do you have grandchildren?

_____

_____

Do you have regular physicals?

_____

_____

Describe the history of your life, your accomplishments, your desires, your disappointments, and
your overall take on how your life has been so far.

_____

_____

What is the best piece of advice you can give to
young people?

_____

_____

Online Resources

Now that you have reached the end of the book, you are at the beginning of the new you. This book contains so much information that it is likely you will put in down and pick it many times over. Whenever you need a little advice, a reminder, a mood boost, whatever it might be to help you continue to *Eat Well, Live Well, Age Well*, this treasure trove of information will be here waiting for you.

Below is a list of links that you can go to for information and to keep you connected.

> For more information about **Patricia Greenberg, The Fitness Gourmet**, and this book, go to www.eatwelllivewellagewell.com

All aspects of aging well

> For **general information and support on aging** your "go to" is AARP, the American Association of Retired Persons. Their stated mission is "to empower people to choose how they live as they age." www.aarp.org

> **National Council on Aging's Center for Healthy Aging.** This non-profit service and advocacy organization serves as a voice for older adults. It brings together nonprofit organizations, businesses, and government to develop creative solutions to assist seniors with their health, living arrangements, jobs and work benefits, and how to remain active in their communities. www.ncoa.org

> **The National Institute on Aging.** The aging process can be daunting. This arm of the National Institutes of Health supports research on aging, illness, and special problems of older people. Its free publications cover a broad variety of topics on aging. www.nia.nih.gov

To learn about how to live like you are in the Blue Zones:
www.bluezones.com/

Emotional well-being and mental health are very important as we age. Reach out for help to reduce stress! The Anxiety and Depression Association of America provide learning tools and advocate to increase awareness and improve diagnosis, treatment, and cure of anxiety disorders.
www.adaa.org

If you would like help addressing **addictive behaviors**, consider reaching out to the various "anonymous" programs, including:
AA (Alcoholics Anonymous)
www.aa.org
Al-Anon (for loved ones of Alcoholics)
www.al-anon.or
Narcotics Anonymous
www.na.org
Overeaters Anonymous (see below)
www.oa.org
Gamblers Anonymous, Spenders Anonymous, Adult Children of Alcoholics, and many more. You can search them all online and find understanding support from a welcoming fellowship.

Your heart, lungs and circulatory systems are what keep you going. American Heart Association, The American Stroke Association, and The American Lung Association are affiliate organizations with a wealth of information on Cardiovascular and Pulmonary health. Free publications are available both in print and online to keep current with the latest research. The American Diabetes Association also provides helpful health information.
www.heart.org
www.strokeassociation.org

www.lungusa.org
www.diabetes.org

Food and Nutrition information can be very confusing. I recommend The National Institute of Health/healthy-eating website. It is comprehensive and very helpful.
www.nia.nih.gov/health/healthy-eating

If you need group support to help you keep on track, I highly recommend Weight Watchers. They provide excellent learning tools for eating healthy for life.
www.weightwatchers.com

OverEaters Anonymous. Whether food is a crutch or a full blown addiction, Twelve Step programs have helped millions of people cope. OA addresses a wide variety of maladjusted relationships to food, including anorexia and bulimia as well as overeating.
www.oa.org

Free food and fitness trackers. Research has shown that those who track their food and exercise are more likely to stick with a program and see results than those who do not. Try one of these:
www.sparkpeople.com
www.loseit.com
www.myfitnesspal.com
www.carbmanager.com

Topics of **fitness** are often geared toward the young and athletic. Here are two of my favorites for ages 50 and up that provide information and locations to pursue your fitness goals. You can also go to WebMD for more info on the benefits of exercise as we age with some great tips on how to get started.

American council on Exercise (ACE). American Council on Exercise is a nonprofit that promotes fitness and offers a wide range of education

materials for both consumers and professionals. There is also a referral service if you are looking for certified fitness trainers in your area.
www.acefitness.org

Silver Sneakers is for older adults of all fitness levels and is covered by secondary insurance for Medicare eligible consumers.
www.silversneakers.com

Arthritis If you are experiencing swelling, pain, stiffness and decreased range of motion in the areas around your joints, its likely to be arthritis.
www.arthritis.org

Chair fitness exercises for resistance and balance are:
www.verywellfit.com/seated-upper-body-workout-1231439
www.vivehealth.com/blogs/resources/chair-exercises-for-seniors

Chair Yoga exercises can be found at:
www.healthline.com/health/fitness-exercise/chair-yoga-for-seniors#1
www.verywellfit.com/chair-yoga-poses-3567189
www.doyouyoga.com/6-benefits-of-chair-yoga-8-poses-to-get-you-started/

Shockingly, most of the websites about "appearance as we age" have to do with selling us products or services to improve our appearance, rather than addressing how to accept or enhance our looks as the years go by. The **body positive** movement is a godsend for people looking to find sites and blogs that empower us, rather than shame us. Find the encouragement and support of your tribe at:
www.bodyimagemovement.com/about/
www.seasonedtimes.com/body-image-and-aging.html
www.themirnavator.com/category/the-blog

Coping With Clutter. Check out information by Marie Kondo, the author of The Life changing Magic of Tidying Up" and Margareta Magnusson, author of "The Gentle Art of Swedish Death Cleaning", by as well as other ways to clear the decks to add energy to your years.
www.konmari.com
www.buzzfeed.com/gyanyankovich/what-is-swedish-death-cleaning
www.flylady.net

Getting old should be fun

Suddenly Senior. Top-ranked website with over 4,000 pages of humor, nostalgia, senior advocacy and useful information. Weekly updates! You can also subscribe to their daily e-zine for everyone over 50 who feels way too young to be old.
www.suddenlysenior.com

Senior Planet "celebrates aging by sharing information and resources that support aging with attitude." Topics include news, health, sex and dating, senior style, travel and entertainment.
www.seniorplanet.org

Boomercafe. The original place for storytelling and smart journalism by baby boomers with active, youthful lifestyles. Find your peers at
www.boomercafe.com

Caregiver support when you're handling the care for your own aging parents or loved ones is available.
www.caregiverstress.com

Resources for end of life care and arrangements

Eldercare is a service of the U.S. Administration on Aging, that can help you find local resources ranging from in-home care, meal assistance, housing alternatives, home repair and legal advice. The

locator also lists state and local agencies on aging.
www.eldercare.gov

Other **housing assistance** websites include
www.seniorly.com
www.aplaceformom.com
for information about assisted living, memory
care, and more.

The Conversation Project provides questions and
conversation starters that people can use to enter
into difficult conversations about what they would
like for end of life care.
www.theconversationproject.com

Wills, Trust and Probate. Here is a great site to set up
all of your own wills, trusts and probate. It is comforting knowing that your wishes will be legally
binding, this granted, after you die.
www.nolo.com/legal-encyclopedia/wills-trusts-estates

Advance Directives. National Hospice and Palliative
Care Organization. has state-specific advance directives that you can obtain online for free. You
have the option of updating these as often as you
wish, so that they are always current.
www.caringinfo.org/AdvanceDirectives.

Funerals. The details for many services are planned
through religious organizations, such as churches,
synagogues, or mosques, and affiliated funeral
homes. There are also national providers such as
the Neptune Society
www.neptunesociety.com
At any of these, preplanning is always much more
cost-effective than trying to arrange details at the
last minute, when everyone is upset and not thinking clearly.

Living Funerals. Read this article for some ideas and
suggestions about how to host a party to bring
together all your friends and relatives before you

die rather than afterwards, so you can be there and share stories, too.
www.nextavenue.org/strange-but-true-some-now-hold-their-funerals-before-dying

Financial Planning and Estate Planning. Getting your financial house in order will make your later years peaceful. The stress we carry due to financial woes makes life miserable and is dangerous to your health. Get your retirement, senior health insurance, savings, investments, and any extra income in place so you can relax.

Social Security
www.ssa.gov

Medicare
www.medicare.gov

IRA, Roth Ira
www.irs.gov/retirement-plans/
individual-retirement-arrangements-iras

Find support to deal with the aging process through your faith community or other shared interest groups. One of dozens — probably hundreds — where you can seek spiritual inspiration is www.beliefnet.com

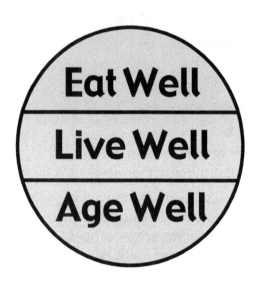

About the Author

Patricia Greenberg, The Fitness Gourmet

Ushering in a new era of bite-sized livable health, nutrition and fitness solutions, Patricia Greenberg, The Fitness Gourmet has 30 years of experience as a Nutritionist, Chef, and Wellness educator. She continues to lives a healthy lifestyle in an often chaotic world through good food and attainable fitness.

Patricia has "Run the Run", completing 20 marathons and 115 half marathons both in the US and internationally. She also enjoys the unique sport of tower climbing and has conquered The Empire State Building, The World Trade Center Freedom Tower, US Bank building, AON building, and the Hancock Tower.

Patricia is the author of four books, and a frequent guest expert on national television and radio programs. She has a special interest in enhancing the education of the general public, providing accurate health information to today's savvy consumer.

Patricia has a BS in Nutrition and Food Science, a Culinary Arts Degree, is an ACE Certified Trainer in Sports Nutrition and Senior Fitness, a Certified "Silver Sneakers" instructor, and a volunteer educator for "Dementia Friends LA."

For more information and to purchase books
www.thefitnessgourmet.com

Made in USA - North Chelmsford, MA
1033609_9780578602721
12.09.2019 1225